Who Owns Your Health?

Who Owns Your Health?

Medical Professionalism and the Market State

Thomas Faunce, B.Med., Ph.D.

The Johns Hopkins University Press | Baltimore

First published in Australia in 2007 by the University of New South Wales Press Ltd

First published in the United States in 2008 by the Johns Hopkins University Press
9 8 7 6 5 4 3 2 1

The Johns Hopkins University Press
2715 North Charles Street
Baltimore, Maryland 21218-4363
www.press.jhu.edu

Library of Congress Control Number: 2007932638

ISBN 13: 978-0-8018-8843-4
ISBN 10: 0-8018-8843-3

Design: Joshua Leui'i
Printer: Griffin Press

CONTENTS

WITHDRAWN

PREFACE

This book outlines the basic principles of moral philosophy, bioethics, health law and international human rights relevant to global health care and medical professionalism. It goes further than similar texts, however, in terms of rigorously promoting critical analysis of the interaction of these systems with conscience. This is achieved through the conceptual device of imagining the relevant consequences of health policy-makers implementing a strategy to fully privatise health service delivery and access to medical technologies around the world.

Powerful forces, as we shall see, appear to support such a strategy. This book investigates whether, even if only partially realised, it might encourage the ethos of the health professionals and policy-makers who staff and govern our major health care institutions to substantially reflect the attitudes and conceptions of the corporate world. It then seeks to understand whether this might not only erode crucial social capital, but remove one of the last and most influential bulwarks of expert critical thinking in the public good.

Advocates of greater privatisation in health care (or sceptics about its deleterious effects) might argue that an institutional ethos accentuating profit-making is not necessarily incompatible with one of community service. They might claim that there will always be a tension between values developed in medical education and the practical requirements of efficient employment and service delivery. They might likewise assert that in terms of standards supervision, patient safety, community benefit and doctor welfare, it matters little who is paying medical professionals or health policy-makers. The global expansion of privatised health care, they could maintain, will probably promote greater competition for quality and safety targets, more transparency (at least by governments), a greater range of experience for trainees and more consistent care even for the underprivileged through the consistent application of managed care protocols and statutory obligations. It is unconscionable, they would state, for tribes of community activists to criticise benevolent industries that strive to serve the public interest through the research and development of innovative technologies which generate increased financial returns for shareholders and sustain economic prosperity.[1]

Those studying the methods involved in corporate takeovers of public goods are likely to be familiar with these types of promises and assertions about the value of privatisation. Their generally well-resourced and influential proponents typically have a variety of objectives, apart from the creation of just and sustainable policy, in criticising any opposing point of view as involving bias, emotion, paranoia and even conspiracy theories, no matter how well intentioned, researched or balanced the presentation of such views is.

This text seeks to move this debate beyond such polarised positions. It strives to explore, objectively and with due respect for all relevant points of view, the question of whether (and to what extent) a dominant ethos of profit-making in health care is indeed compatible, in the long term, with one of community service. In doing this, it examines the role that professional conscience and virtue, on the one hand, and pecuniary gain, on the other, have had in developing the canons of professionalism, and may yet play in renegotiating the place of the corporate health care sector in a global social contract. It also investigates the regulatory strategies by which both the advantages of corporate competition and important global public goods in health care may be preserved in and beyond the age of the market state. This text does not investigate a governance movement beyond markets but how they can become more focused on sustainability and conscience.

This work, appropriately, draws upon interviews the author conducted in 2005 with the public-funded pharmaceutical cost-effectiveness experts on the Australian Pharmaceutical Benefits Advisory Committee (PBAC) and with senior executives of all major pharmaceutical companies based in Australia. This research was funded by an Australian Research Council (ARC) grant to investigate the impact of the Australia–United States Free Trade Agreement (AUSFTA) on Australian medicines policy. Interviews were also carried out with pharmaceutical cost-effectiveness regulators and industry representatives in Canada, the United States, South Korea and China.

This book builds upon a variety of monograph chapters and refereed articles I have published since 2000. In particular, it sets into a particular context and amplifies arguments about normative interactions between bioethics, health law and human rights that I first outlined in *Pilgrims in Medicine* (where such concepts were personified as acting over the course of their careers). I use several examples and constructions I've used before, but with, I hope, greater clarity and precision. Case studies at the end of each chapter are designed to crystallise the conceptual issues raised upon practical and identifiable dilemmas in the lives of individuals.

My sincere thanks to John Elliot, Heather Cam and the other staff at UNSW Press and to Sarah Shrubb for her insightful assistance at the editing stage.

ABBREVIATIONS

UDHR: United Nations, Universal Declaration of Human Rights, adopted 10 December 1948, GA Res 217A (III), UN Doc A/810 (1948) 71.

ICCPR: United Nations, International Covenant on Civil and Political Rights, adopted 16 December 1966, entry into force 23 March 1976. GA Res 2200A (XXI) 21, UN GAOR, Supp (No. 16) 52, UN Doc A/6316 (1966), 999 UNTS 17, repr (1967) 6 Int Legal Materials 368. 144 states parties.

ICESCR: United Nations, International Covenant on Economic, Social and Cultural Rights adopted 16 December 1966, entry into force 3 January 1976. GA Res 2200A (XXI), UN Doc A/6316 (1966) 993 UNTS 3, repr (1967) 6 *Int Legal Materials* 360. 142 states parties.

GENOCIDE CONVENTION: United Nations, Convention on the Prevention and Punishment of the Crime of Genocide, adopted 9 December 1948, entry into force 12 January 1951. (1948) 78 *UNTS* 277. 130 states parties.

TORTURE CONVENTION: United Nations, Convention Against Torture and Other Cruel, Inhuman or Degrading Treatment or Punishment, adopted 10 December 1984, entry into force 26 June 1987, GA Res 39/46, 39 UN GAOR, Supp (No 51), UN Doc A/39/51 (1984) 197, repr (1985) 24 *Int Legal Materials* 535. 118 states parties.

RACIAL DISCRIMINATION CONVENTION: United Nations, International Convention on the Elimination of all Forms of Racial Discrimination, adopted 21 December 1965, entry into force 4 January 1969. (1965) 660 *UNTS* 195, repr (1966) 5 *Int Legal Materials* 352. 155 states parties.

CEDAW: United Nations, Convention on the Elimination of all Forms of Discrimination Against Women, adopted 18 December 1979, entry into force 3 September 1981,

GA Res 34/180, 34 UNGAOR, Supp (no 46),
UN Doc A/34/46 (1979) 193, (1979) 1249 *UNTS* 13,
repr (1980) 19 *Int Legal Materials* 33. 165 states parties.

CROC: Convention on the Rights of the Child, adopted
20 November 1989, entry into force 2 September 1990,
GA Res 44/25, 44 UNGAOR, Supp (No 49),
UN Doc A/44/49 (1989) 166, repr (1989) 28 *Int Legal
Materials* 1448. 191 states parties.

ECHR: European Convention for the Protection of Human Rights
and Fundamental Freedoms, signed 4 November 1950, entry
into force 3 September 1953, 213 *UNTS* 221. ETS 5 (1950).
41 states parties.

CONVENTION ON HUMAN RIGHTS AND BIOMEDICINE: Council of
Europe, Convention for the Protection of Human Rights and
Dignity of the Human Being with Regard to the Application
of Biology and Medicine, signed 4 April 1997.
ETS 164 (1997).

UDHGHR: United Nations Economic, Social and Cultural
Organisation (UNESCO), Universal Declaration on the
Human Genome and Human Rights,
signed 11 November 1997.

UDBHR: UNESCO, Universal Declaration on Bioethics and
Human Rights.

GATS: World Trade Organization, General Agreement on Trade
and Services.

TRIPs: World Trade Organization, Trade-Related Intellectual
Property Rights Agreement.

DOHA DECLARATION: World Trade Organization, 2001, Doha
Declaration on the TRIPs Agreement and Public Health.
WT/MIN/(01)/Dec/W/2.

*To Benedict 'Ben' Chifley, TC 'Tommy' Douglas and Nye Bevan,
who reminded doctors about their professional ideals, and for
those supporting conscience and public goods in global health care.*

DECLARATION OF GENEVA

AT THE TIME OF BEING ADMITTED AS A MEMBER OF THE MEDICAL PROFESSION:

I SOLEMNLY PLEDGE to consecrate my life to the service of humanity;

I WILL GIVE to my teachers the respect and gratitude that is their due;

I WILL PRACTISE my profession with conscience and dignity;

THE HEALTH OF MY PATIENT will be my first consideration;

I WILL RESPECT the secrets that are confided in me, even after the patient has died;

I WILL MAINTAIN by all the means in my power, the honour and the noble traditions of the medical profession;

MY COLLEAGUES will be my sisters and brothers;

I WILL NOT PERMIT considerations of age, disease or disability, creed, ethnic origin, gender, nationality, political affiliation, race, sexual orientation, social standing or any other factor to intervene between my duty and my patient;

I WILL MAINTAIN the utmost respect for human life;

I WILL NOT USE my medical knowledge to violate human rights and civil liberties, even under threat;

I MAKE THESE PROMISES solemnly, freely and upon my honour.

1

THE
CORPORATE
CHALLENGE
TO
MEDICAL
PROFESSIONALISM

I. Leadership in an increasingly privatised global health care system

§i. Consecrated to the service of humanity?

Medicine, like law, is often considered a prime example of a profession. As professions, these occupations were traditionally held to involve elements not present in, for example, a trade or business. Their members were deemed to have special skills or learning, whose development and use was rewarded by a state-sanctioned monopoly. Crucially distinctive, however, was the expectation that any resultant acquisition of wealth remained incidental to a fundamental ethos of community service. The private ambitions and personal acquisitions of a society's professionals, their ability to function as power elites, with the capacity to influence bureaucracies and political leaders, were tolerated as a privilege, on trust that they would be subordinated to a compensating facilitation of public good. Managers, policy-makers and corporate executives involved in health care have a less substantial historical background as professionals with a primary service ethos.

In this book I intend to explore some consequences of the hypothesis that corporate interests may soon be dominating not only the practical provision and regulation of health care but, increasingly, the ethos of health professionals worldwide. One resultant risk is of tension developing between the basic virtues and principles of medical professionalism and the achievement of organisational goals related to maximising shareholder and managerial profit in a global free market.

I argue that it matters how doctors, industry executives, health managers, lawyers and policy-makers think about such a globally privatised vision of health care. Such reflection may impact strongly on the quality and equity of health care delivery, as well as on general social governance values and ideals.

I propose to consider what should be the underlying principles whose consistent application will shape the professional leadership roles in global heath care of doctors, industry representatives, managers and policy-makers. This initially will be done through an exploration of themes emerging from the historical origins of medical professionalism. I then try to construct and defend a particular theory about the kind of regulation of health care professionalism that may be best suited to improving outcomes for all relevant stakeholders beyond the era of the market state. This perspective, a long-term one, reflects my concern that the inevitable transformation of the market state towards greater protection of social capital and public goods in areas such as health care facilitates, rather than inhibits, the emergence of a more genuinely cosmopolitan, egalitarian and sustainable global civilisation.

§ii. *Practise with conscience and dignity?*

As we'll see, the visionary agenda for humanity based on human rights, fundamental freedoms and respect for inherent human dignity owes much to ancient medical ethics.[1] Yet many would now strongly deny any sustained or coordinated role of doctors – either in the past or today – as moral arbiters, exemplars of conscience and respecters of human dignity. What is there, they might ask, in the training or expertise of the physician, surgeon, intensivist, anaesthetist, general practitioner or medical researcher, for example, which would justify any particular claim to moral authority or insight concerning society as a whole?

In his plays *The Seagull*, *Uncle Vanya* and *The Three Sisters*, Russian playwright and physician Anton Chekhov explored, as a subsidiary theme, the essence of medical professionalism and leadership. He examined what happens morally and spiritually to a doctor who ignores conscience in his making of clinical judgments. Dr Dorn in *The Seagull*, for example, is a 55-year-old bachelor who has so detached himself from the virtues of empathy and compassion that he escapes intimacy and bursts into meaningless song, or takes valerian, whenever conversation threatens to become substantial. Dr Astrov, in *Uncle Vanya*, saturates himself with vodka and refuses marriage, to dull the emotional torture of remembering his professional failures. Dr Chebutykin, in *The Three Sisters*, likewise indulges himself with endless rationalisation, fantasy and flirting, to hide his lack of vocational commitment. When the nearby villagers plead for his assistance during a fire, he says, 'in my heart and soul … I felt twisted, corrupt, ugly … I went and got drunk'.

Misfits such as those described by Chekhov are present in any profession, but, as we'll see, there is now growing evidence that from the 1970s onwards, patients in developed nations have become far less likely to regard doctors generally as social leaders. They seem less tolerant of any perceived a lack of medical understanding, insensitive or inaccurate delivery of medical material risk information, or lack of professional interest, care and motivation. They, or their relatives, appear to more readily threaten litigation (rather than merely lodge official complaints), seek second opinions, and transfer to 'alternative' medical therapies. Upset patients frequently assert such 'rights' even when no physical or mental injury has been inflicted and no legal rules have been clearly broken by their physicians.

In developed nations, many patients perceive doctors as part of a lucrative, socially privileged subculture that is pushing health service consumers into complex, managerially directed, cost-saving diagnostic and therapeutic 'pathways'. They experience great difficulty in acquiring information about the relative competence of physicians and surgeons. Increasing numbers report feeling suspicious of, or estranged from the values of their physicians. Others, of course, are greatly appreciative of access to life-saving new health technologies, pharmaceuticals and medical devices. Valuing their health and that of their family, they are prepared to pay appropriate insurance premiums to obtain access to high quality care. Many of the profession's leaders – and even some patient advocacy groups, no doubt – will actually support the full global privatisation of health care.

Nomenclature changes such as those categorising patients as 'consumers' and doctors as 'providers' have been promoted recently by health advocacy and statutory complaints organisations as useful for balancing legal power in that relationship. Such terminological revisions, however, arguably also highlight a fundamental confusion about the values of contemporary medicine. Will calling a patient a 'consumer' in all clinical settings, for example, undermine the traditional professional protections of patients?

Such concerns, and many others explored in this book, have led to a number of international projects to reinvigorate medical professionalism.[2] These projects uniformly emphasise social responsibility, as well as the need for a new 'compact' or moral and social justice 'contract', amongst all relevant stakeholders, particularly government, public, industry, health service managers and patient groups. One hypothesis I wish to explore is that considering such a contract may involve expanding the categories of health professionals and reorganising their service obligations, particularly in relation to global public goods.

One of the qualities of good leadership in the public interest is the capacity to readily discern new factors that are likely to require policy change. Another is the ability to inspire, enunciate and implement a practical program of response, consistent not only with immediate organisational goals, but also with the best ideals of humanity. This book is written in the belief that leaders amongst physicians, industry, health managers, lawyers and policy-makers should accept professional responsibilities to make significant contributions in this important debate.

II. Historical tensions in medical professionalism and health policy

§i. *The vulnerable foundations of medical professionalism*

The following sections will explore the concept of medical professionalism through a variety of historical settings and cultural traditions. The aim is to discern elements likely to shape the nature and function of health care regulation in and beyond what I refer to as the age of the market state. 'Market state' is a term I use in this book to refer to governments that have formed a close policy bond with industry, to the extent, in many senses, that their interests are mutually perceived as indistinguishable and superior to any countervailing community concerns. I recognise that this is, in itself, a politically controversial concept. Yet it is intended to be a value-neutral, and realistically objective, descriptor that facilitates rational policy debate in a period of increased interest in health care privatisation. I use the terms 'medical professionalism' and 'health care professionalism' interchangeably, to emphasise both their shared value origins and their broader applicability to the key participants in global health care delivery.

By way of preliminary explanation, the good sought by any regulatory system may be termed a *telos*, and philosophies designed to achieve its maximisation are known as teleological. Many forms of the political and moral philosophy known as utilitarianism, for example, focus on the goal (or *telos*) of encouraging overall community welfare (the greatest good for the greatest number). Deontological theories, in broad terms, support the upholding of key moral and ethical principles for their own sake, or that of the (mostly religious) authority propounding them.

It is intriguing to consider that during the origins of medical professionalism, little practical distinction was made between principles of religion and medical ethics and those of science, then a fledgling discipline. Whether a doctor, for example, should always obey the principle of helping his or her injured neighbour regardless of capacity to pay, whether an apple should consistently follow the rule of falling when released from its twig, or gout be viewed as a divine punishment for the vice of gluttony, were equally matters to be wholly resolved by philosophical or theological speculation. To some extent, as we'll see, the contemporary policy dominance of the ideology described as 'free market fundamentalism' may represent a recrudescence of such pseudo-scientific ideas.

Medicine appears to have been first referred to as a 'profession' or vocation by Scribonius Largus in the first century AD, in his treatise *Compositiones Medicamentorum* (*On Remedies*). The act of 'professing' generally involved standing in a public place and making a commitment, before society, colleagues and the appropriate Divinity, to uphold certain principles of service to the general good. As an expected ceremony at the commencement of a medical career, it made the duties expressed in professional oaths open to public scrutiny and more coherent with the community's traditions.[3] Taking an oath was also a public affirmation that a doctor intended to integrate the profession's foundational ethical principles into his (there were few, if any, female doctors in those days) conscience. It was undoubtedly a leadership gesture.

The humanistic egalitarianism of Scribonius's professionalism, remarkable for its time, appears to have been influenced by Cicero's *De Officiis*. Cicero, writing in the first century BC and heavily influenced by the Greek Stoic philosophers, became renowned for tracing Roman law to principles of reason that were supposedly inherent in all rational human beings. This early connection between so-called natural law jurisprudence and medical professionalism highlights their common focus on generating rules of conduct from universal ideals. In the medieval period, those practising medicine were already seen in two very different ways: as people who had consecrated their lives to either salvation through helping those in need, or a not-so-idealistic quest for exceedingly great profit.

§ii. *The Hippocratic Oath's archaic sensibilities*

Many view the core principles of contemporary medical professionalism as having a necessary, although not sufficient, connection with the culture-neutral values expressed in the *Hippocratic Oath*. This iconic 2500-year-old statement of foundational professional virtues and principles was written on the Greek island of Kos, fragmented, reassembled in Alexandria in 350 BC, and has been transmitted and preserved through the ages along a chain of academic and professional luminaries.

The *Hippocratic Oath* espouses the medical duties not to do harm (non-maleficence), to enter houses only for the good of patients (beneficence), to practise within the bounds of competence and to respect patients' confidences, even after they are dead. It has become a practical manifestation of the natural law position that the best human beings are intrinsically constituted to seek an altruistic good, which manifests here in an egalitarian respect for human dignity remarkable, though not necessarily unique, for its time.

The *Hippocratic Oath* was originally an oath in the true sense, with allegiances sworn in secret to feared deities. Such an oath – like the one made by Hamlet to his father's ghost (or, he fears, the Devil) and that the young prince urges his companions to take on the frosty midnight battlements of Elsinore – encourages obedience in conscience to specific principles or rules. It does this by linking those principles or rules to a credible threat of supernatural sanction. Oath-taking frequently sets the scene for morally instructive later conflict between fated circumstance and the protagonists' commitment to principles thus affirmed as critical to their life narrative.

The *Hippocratic Oath*, in its original form, contained many encouragements to medical virtue ('I will preserve the purity of my life and art') focused on establishing a doctor's career as a public good, an item of social capital. Yet the first stated ethical rule of the *Hippocratic Oath* was actually that the doctor owed foremost loyalty to his brethren and teachers, rather than to the patient. Hippocrates stated elsewhere in his writings that the doctor's relationship to the patient 'must be that of the person in command to one who obeys'. Respect for patient autonomy was not mentioned. Slaves and women also had an extremely problematic place within the tenets of the *Hippocratic Oath*. It has been accused of accentuating a privileged guild mentality, a concept of clinical medicine as a gentleman's club.

The *Hippocratic Oath*, despite acquiring secretive, sexist, paternalistic and elitist elements (largely derived from its historical circumstances), has remained a core document in medical professionalism. Its modern restatement, as the *Geneva Declaration* (revised frequently since 1948 and reproduced at the front of this work), still makes doctors swear an oath to develop and maintain foundational virtues: to consecrate their life to the service of humanity, to practise their profession with 'conscience and dignity' and to make the health of the patient their first consideration. Most medical graduation oaths now use the *Declaration of Geneva*. Islamic schools utilise the *Declaration of Kuwait*.[4] Some contemporary medical students create their own graduating oath, viewing it as a seed of hope that a primary commitment to service rather than profit may remain a dominant focus of their careers. Increasing numbers, however, in debt from expensive basic and specialist degrees and necessarily aspiring to lucrative private sector employment to support their families, see such oath-taking as a meaningless and archaic ritual. Corporate executives, managers and policy-makers involved in contemporary health care currently do not generally take an oath upon assuming their duties.

Hippocrates, like tragically flawed Hamlet, overly twisted by conscience and courage, has become an archetypal figure in Western civilisation, one whose stature relates to the aggregation of ideals that cluster about his name. Time and again in the great regulatory crises that have beset clinical medicine, Hippocrates' *Oath* has been reverentially referred to as exemplifying the most respected virtues of the profession. Yet the *Hippocratic Oath* should undoubtedly be regarded as an incomplete, evolving, aspirational (rather than perfect) statement of the virtues and principles inherent in medical professionalism.

When Paracelsus ('surpassing Celsus'), the *nom de guerre* of Theophrastus Philippus Aureolus Bombastus von Hohenheim, led his medieval students to turn from Hippocrates and the authoritative medical texts of Galen and learn the truth of disease from observation and experience, he was not denigrating the ethical core of the *Hippocratic Oath*. Rather, he was enflamed by its very sentiments to attack and reform a version of medical professionalism that was producing a 'miserable art' that seemed to mostly result in 'killing and laming'. One important issue that any new social contract on global health will have to face is the extent to which, in an era beyond that of the market state, the *Hippocratic Oath* can or should retain a prominent role in shaping ideals of health care professionalism.

§iii. *Islamic, Buddhist and other non-Christian traditions*

The *Hippocratic Oath* has traditionally played a large part in discussions about the normative foundations of medical professionalism and health policy. Yet foundational principles of medical ethics – such as that requiring humanitarian egalitarianism in diagnosis and treatment – were not reaffirmed only in Graeco-Roman-Christian culture. Likewise, belief that humans have a non-physical soul (or conscience) appears to be a cultural universal that saturates all early records of medical professionalism. Such common cross-cultural professional understandings are explored here to suggest fruitful areas of research and because they may affirm, as will subsequently be discussed, a socially unifying role for professional conscience within a fully privatised global health care system.

Much more work could be done, for example, on assessing the extent to which early Arabic medical ethics oaths and texts emphasised the primary importance of the physician's purity of virtue, conscience and soul.[5] Hippocrates' contribution to medical professionalism should be assessed alongside that of great physicians in the Muslim tradition, such as Avicenna (Ibn Sina). These doctors were titled *hakim*, a term denoting society's expectation they would strive for career excellence in a manner involving practical wisdom and moral leadership. A valuable assessment could be made, for example, of the normative importance to general Islamic society of endowments setting up charitable hospitals. Many of these, for example, state that doctors were expected to treat male and female, rich and poor, of any race or religion, with large or small illnesses, equally and, often, without cost to the patient.

Medical professionals of all nations should be aware that these traditions are reflected in that authoritative modern statement of Islamic medical ethics, the *Declaration of Kuwait*. This requires doctors to focus on service (*ummah*) relieving the suffering of the needy, be they 'near or far, virtuous or sinner, friend or enemy'.[6] Those doubting the present relevance of such professional ideals (alongside the foundational social virtue of *taqwa*, which means 'righteousness', 'piety' or 'God-consciousness') in Islamic cultures should study the idealistic and courageous activities of Doctors for Iraq, a non-governmental organisation under the intense pressures of a contemporary armed conflict zone.

In contemporary Muslim discourse (and this appears increasingly also the case in Western democracies influenced by the Christian Right), the moral, ethical and legal rules that underpin health policy are regularly calibrated against religious principles. This suggests that in such countries, agreement about the foundational principles of medical professionalism should evolve from a discourse amongst policy-makers that balances commitments to socially endogenous religious virtues (such as *taqwa* or 'loving thine enemies') and cosmopolitan virtues and principles from international human rights (such as 'respect for human dignity') with principles (such as 'recognition of pharmaceutical innovation') emerging from the free market ideology underpinning certain bilateral trade agreements and those of the World Trade Organization (WTO).

There is no generally accepted traditional Jewish code of medical ethics, but leading physicians in that culture, such as Moses Maimonides, should receive greater emphasis in contemporary discussions of medical professionalism.[7] The crucial social field of action for uniquely Jewish conceptions of medical professionalism is likely to remain the Israeli-Palestinian conflict, particularly due to the potential for it (if unresolved) to promote terrorism and undermine world peace.

It is similarly important to emphasise that the classical Chinese equivalent of the *Hippocratic Oath* appears to have been a parchment entitled *On the Absolute Sincerity of Great Physicians* by Sun Simiao. Physicians were here requested to cultivate the virtues of compassion, pity and egalitarian treatment:

A Great Physician should not pay attention to status, wealth or age; neither should he question whether the particular [patient] is attractive or unattractive, whether he [or she] is an enemy or friend, whether he [or she] is a Chinese or foreigner, or finally, whether he [or she] is uneducated or educated. He should meet everyone on equal ground. He should always act as if he were thinking of his close relatives.[8]

Confucius considered the virtues of loyalty (*chung*), being trustworthy in words (*xin*) and acting with consideration or empathy for others (*shu*) to be of fundamental importance to those in professional and public life. Like Aristotle, he encouraged personal equilibrium and harmony gradually acquired through the virtue of loyalty (*zhong yong*) to principles supporting social good, as more important than fanatical obedience to any human master. Confucius's 'highest' virtue, *ren*, resembles the paean to altruism expressed in the secular categorical imperative of Kant, or the 'neighbour' component of Christ's prime commandment. The literal translation of *ren* is 'two-man-mindedness' or 'mindfulness of the other person'. The *traveaux préparatoires* of documents such as the *Universal Declaration of Human Rights* show that the drafters explicitly recognised the association between 'conscience' in Article 1 and the Chinese virtue *ren*.

The people and rulers of many contemporary Asian states (particularly China) appear to show more commitment in their public health policies to free market fundamentalist ideology than to such professional and social virtues and principles. The picture is made even more complex, however, because the citizens of so many nations (regardless of prior traditions) are now embracing fanatical forms of Muslim and Christian faiths, or indeed the mass media-indoctrinated consumerist belief that ultimate happiness resides in unlimited purchasing power.

In Buddhism, individual virtues such as compassion and equanimity (also traditionally central to medical professionalism) are regarded as a means to the ultimate goal of a well-considered human life. This requires constant mental equanimity (*nibbana*), achieved through a lifetime of compassionate work undertaken with detachment from the selfish possessiveness and dissatisfaction (*dukkha*) that results from most attempts by human beings to impose material and emotional stability and permanence upon the flux of reality. In philosophical terms, Buddhist ethics uses the term 'suffering' in a much broader sense than might be universally applicable in medical professionalism. Veracity, non-injury to life, the impropriety of interrupting another's *kamma*, and compassion are fundamental virtues and principles from the Buddhist tradition that have particular relevance to medical professionalism.

Specialised *zen* Buddhist forms of philosophy, art and literature traditionally emphasise a morality based upon a transformation of character through meditatively trained insight into the relation between a non-physical self (or soul) and the world. The capacity to still and focus the mind for minutes at a time is conceived of as assisting a more positive coalescence between social and personal consciousness and ideals. The foundational social virtue of *zen* Buddhism appears to be *wa*, rather than justice or fairness. *Wa*, encompassing conciliation, concord, unity, harmony and reconciliation, naturally resides at the heart of Japanese bioethics. Interestingly, however, it was not to the foundational social virtue of *wa* that judges of the Tokyo High Court and Japanese Supreme Court referred when they were trying to discern fundamental principles in 'hard' cases concerning legislative discrimination against illegitimate children. Rather, they sought jurisprudential coherence with international human rights.[9]

Buddhism, with its sceptical relation to God but mystical affirmation of a non-physical soul, is increasingly popular in contemporary global society. Such meditative philosophies have yet to become consistently successful drivers for social welfare policies and legislation in the way Christianity has in the past. Yet they appear to be gaining legitimacy from discoveries in modern science, including quantum physics, of new relationships between consciousness and matter. They could play an important role in peacefully moving beyond the consumerist materialism promoted in market state ideology.

In traditional India, probably only the pharmacological Ayurveda system of medicine had no express ties to a spiritual or religious practice which encouraged virtue in the healer. The *Oath of the Hindu Physician* (327 BC), stated, 'do the sick no harm, not even in thought'. The

Caraka Samhita, a compendium of the sage Caraka, praises the virtuous physician who is 'courteous, wise, self-disciplined, and a master of his subject'. It contains an *Oath of Initiation* which requires a medical student to be celibate, speak the truth, observe a strict vegetarian diet, be free of envy, never carry weapons and remain pledged to the relief of suffering in his patients, while never abandoning or taking sexual advantage of them. Hindu medical students were generally expected to be chaperoned to the patient's home and to respect the confidentiality of professionally disclosed information. Such ideals and their historical associations appear quaint to many current Indian medical students, who, upon graduation, are likely to seek jobs in developed nations, or obtain employment in local biotech research and development clusters, or state-of-the-art private hospitals.

In folk and aboriginal cultures, the virtue of a medical practitioner was often recognised as a therapeutic agent in itself. Practices such as prolonged fasting, prayer and meditation during a socially isolated idealistic vision quest were therefore traditionally acknowledged as part of the healer's training. This has many valuable similarities with what is known as the Western natural law tradition, particularly Thomas Aquinas's view of the immanence in both reality and objective value of a segment of eternal law discernible by human reason searching for coherence with an ideal. These societies provide many valuable lessons about the worth of simple, personal concepts of the sacred achieved through local craft work. Yet by the time young men and women from many such societies have completed training in scientific medicine, few wish to remain in the unstable political and social circumstances, the corruption and violence, of their native 'failed' states. The role of the free market policies of the World Bank, the International Monetary Fund (IMF), the WTO and multinational corporations in precipitating such a knowledge drain will be explored later in this book.

§iv. *Medical science, the social contract and professional etiquette*

From the 1600s, advances in scientific understanding began to shape theories of governance in both general social relations and the medical profession. The medical profession's gradually increasing allegiance to scientific truth was destined to become a powerful legitimising force behind its social power.

In 1628, William Harvey published *Exercitatio Anatomica de Motu Cordis et Sanguinis in Animalibus*. Harvey's famous physiological insight concerning the circular and ceaseless impulsion of blood occurred in the same period as Galileo's (1564–1642) understanding that, in the absence of all forces (including gravity and friction), a body will continue moving indefinitely in a straight line at a constant velocity. It was also contemporary with Descartes' still influential argument that human beings must possess a non-physical component of identity (the soul or conscience), because a thinker cannot rationally deny his or her own existence (but is able to doubt any related role of brain or body).

Such new knowledge became a backdrop to Thomas Hobbes' (1588–1679) theory that the ideal form of governance for a society could be deduced from a series of elementary propositions. Chief amongst these was the claim that human beings individually and collectively were naturally set in motion by selfish emotions and desires that sought to avoid death and suffering and maximise enjoyment. Yet uncontrolled pursuit of individual desires causes citizens constant insecurity, and allows little assurance of peace and safety. Such anarchy resembles the proliferation of frictive forces that retards progress of an object set in motion. It must be prevented by a powerful ruler. This was the Leviathan, who, by mutual agreement of citizens, was accorded power to enforce laws. John Locke and Jean-Jacques Rousseau extended Hobbes' notion of legal authority granted to a powerful ruler under a social contact: to laws, derived by reason from the very nature of humanity, that supported both communal good and the inherent rights of individuals.

This idea of a social contract became a useful focal point for policy development in many nations. One solution involved the creation of constitutions that granted citizens inalienable rights assigned amongst each other, equitably, by fairly administered laws; inequality would only be tolerated if it resulted in compensating benefits for all. Aspects of social contract analysis were developed as a philosophy and policy doctrine known as utilitarianism by Jeremy Bentham and John Stuart

Mill, and as an economic theory supporting the 'invisible hand' of market forces by Adam Smith.

The ideals of public service in the *Hippocratic Oath* were increasingly viewed as promises constituting one half of a social contract, the consideration for which was medical practitioners' lucrative monopoly position. And virtue, conscience and the soul, emphasised implicitly in the *Hippocratic Oath*, were increasingly relegated by the profession to the category of dubiously valuable non-scientific, quasi-superstitious notions.

The nation state was being developed at this time, both practically, through conquest and nationalist propaganda, and as a political and legal concept. It began to appear on maps: geographical areas indicated the existence of, and the land lived on by, particular human societies that were united – as Hobbes predicted and as John Austin's later doctrine of positivism would specify – by common habitual obedience to the laws of a single sovereign. The *Treaty of Westphalia* (1648) affirmed the mutual recognition of states, despite the times being characterised by religious intolerance and warfare. The state acquired international legal personality, privileging the claims of those representing it, much as, it could be argued, senior employment within a multinational corporate entity does in the present era of the market state.

In 1646 Hugo Grotius began to develop the prototype for an international humanitarian law that would bind these abstract entities called states. He proposed that under the natural law (to which all individuals and all states were subject), conscience had a 'judicial power' to be the 'sovereign guide' of human actions; he believed that by despising its admonitions, the human mind was 'stupefied into brutal hardness'.[10] It may be that development beyond the age of the market state will require a similar transformation of understanding about the role of multinational corporations in international governance.

At this time, leaders of the medical profession were engaged in negotiations with representatives of states who desired to secure their populations from the threat of disease (in particular by quarantine against plague) and mistreatment by 'quacks'. Legislation by Henry VIII, for example, which incorporated the Royal College of Physicians in London in 1523 and regulated the professional practice of surgeons, declared its primary purpose to be protecting the public. Clearly, however, the statute was also designed to protect medical incomes from competition.

By the late 1600s, leaders of the empirical approach to clinical practice, such as Thomas Sydenham and Ambrose Paré, were teaching their students to close their precious volumes of Galen and examine each patient as a real person. Sydenham, an openly reverential heir to Hippocrates' ideals, instructed his students to go to the patient's bedside and observe the natural phenomena of diseases, which he believed proliferated consistently, in the way that plants do. 'The selfsame phenomena that you would observe in the sickness of a Socrates,' he wrote, with egalitarian conviction, 'you would observe in the sickness of a simpleton.' This radical change of medical vision saw the patient as an individual with a measure of inherent dignity, rather than as a glimpsed type that could be explained by theoretical and bookish abstractions. Yet leadership such as that exhibited by Sydenham and Paré characteristically took a long time to become uniform practice in the profession.

Physical examination, that most intimate and presently highly legally regulated connection between doctor and patient, only gradually evolved into more than just a cursory glance for fever or spots, an ostentatious observance of the urine, or conventionally restrained palpation of the pulse under bedclothes. Such practices had all too often characterised the care of charlatan physicians similar to the one depicted in the well-known Hogarth painting *Scene with the Quack* (1745). In fact, most doctors, until this time, rarely touched their patients. They viewed such contact as a breach of particular moral principles, and as possibly threatening to the trust on which any alleged cure – and their incomes – depended. The medical profession as a whole was thus prejudiced against percussion of the chest, for example, when Auenbrugger (1722–1809) attempted to introduce it as a diagnostic technique in the late 1700s.

Physical signs of illness were increasingly being correlated, with greater accuracy, to symptoms and post mortem findings, in the painstakingly studious manner of Dr Lydgate in George Eliot's *Middlemarch*. The laying on of the doctor's hands in the search for diagnostic signs became the prime symbolic motif of the professional ideals inherent in the doctor–patient relationship. Touch, used by doctors for its cognitive and diagnostic yield, became synonymous with a community expectation of foundational professional virtues such as empathy, compassion, trust and loyalty.

Ignaz Semmelweis, a law student before he transferred to medicine, is often held up to contemporary students as an idealistic leader of the medical profession. As House Officer (equivalent to a senior registrar today) in Vienna General Hospital, he became determined to find the cause of high rates of fatal maternal infection in the Obstetric Clinic. He noted that the autopsy of a colleague, who died after accidentally cutting his finger during a post mortem, seemed to reveal the same septic pathology as the women dying of what was then called puerperal fever. Semmelweis hypothesised that medical students and junior doctors who had recently examined either corpses in the morgue or infected surgical wounds could somehow be spreading disease. By imposing chlorine hand-washing guidelines he felt he was affirming his commitment to the foundational virtues and principles of the Hippocratic ideal.

His uncompromising commitment to the professional virtues of respect for scientific truth and loyalty to the relief of patient suffering met with outrage, however, from many of his colleagues. They believed he was unnecessarily undermining lucrative and curative patient trust, as well as the social status of the profession. Semmelweis, in actions that remain the customary response of hospital administrators to whistleblowers, was reprimanded, not reappointed, and thus forced to take another job with less status and pay. His successor abolished his guidelines, calling them 'ridiculous'. The great pathologist Rudolph Virchow spoke out against Semmelweis' ideas at an international conference. Semmelweis wrote to one of his professorial critics in these terms:

> I am linked to you by many pleasant memories, but the groans
> of women dying in child-bed drown out the voice of affection.

Semmelweis ended life greatly disturbed in mind. He was beaten to death by the staff of a mental hospital in which he was incarcerated.[11]

John Locke, philosopher and father figure in the human rights movement, was an English physician and close friend of the esteemed empiricist physician Sydenham. Locke had attended lectures on neuroanatomy given by Thomas Willis, after whom the arterial circle supplying the cerebral hemispheres is named. Locke experienced close professional proximity to patient suffering (one of his famous patients was the first Earl of Shaftesbury, whose hydatid cyst abscess he drained with a silver tube from the liver), coupled with direct clinical encouragement from Sydenham to uphold and apply foundational Hippocratic principles, such as professional egalitarianism. This may have assisted him to affirm the ideal that all rational men should be presumed by policy-makers to have inherent ideals about rights in their minds which they only temporarily abandon, on trust, to a sovereign. Locke stated that a legislature or other ruler which attempts, for example, to arbitrarily dispose of the life, liberty or property of its people breaches fundamental principles of the commonly understood social contract ideal, and so forfeits any 'natural' authority.

That great medical iconoclast and whistleblower of the 17th century, Dr Gideon Harvey, frequently and openly referred to the Royal College of Physicians as 'the eldest quack synagogue'. He derided their public expressions of virtue as a hypocritical, self-serving packaging of principles concerned chiefly with correct etiquette. At this time, as but one example, though some doctors travelled long distances to see patient suffering face to face, as it were, others made diagnoses and offered treatment by post.

As scientific knowledge grew, doctors continued to offer service to the state's utilitarian *telos* through public health endeavours. John Howard (c. 1726–90) and the naval and military physicians James Lind (1716–94), John Pringle (1707–82) and John Haygarth (1740–1827), for instance, campaigned against confined quarters and filthy conditions on ships and in prisons, claiming them to be a cause of typhus. Similar efforts were made with respect to smallpox inoculation. Following the work of Edwin Chadwick in investigating a revision of the *Poor Law*, the first British *Public Health Act* was passed, in 1848. This Act created local boards of health that were responsible for sanitary supervision and inspection, for drainage, water and gas supplies, and for appointing local medical officers of health. Similar legislation followed: the *Nuisance Removal and Disease Prevention (Cholera) Act 1848*, the *Sewers Act 1848*, the *Interments Act 1852* and the *Water Act 1852*.

The work of John Simon as Britain's first chief medical administrator culminated in the *Sanitary Act* 1866. Simon believed that the state's obligation was to ensure, by legal regulation, the 'physical conditions of existence', which included sufficient supply of sanitary housing, wholesome, unadulterated food and drugs, the control of epidemic diseases and state regulation of qualified medical practice.

This was the social and historical context in which Norwegian playwright Henrik Ibsen's fictional Dr Stockman became an 'enemy of the people' when he claimed that the baths on which a town's economy was based were actually a source of bacterial infection. Quarantine laws implemented by medical professionals became a notorious source of cruelty towards and degradation of patients, an issue French author Albert Camus dealt with through his description of Dr Rieux in *The Plague*. Both these examples have obvious resonance with a fully privatised global health care system seeking to respond to threats of bioterrorism and emergent infectious disease pandemics.

§v. Christian leadership of medical professionalism

By the late 19th century, many leaders of the medical profession began to express the view that the *Hippocratic Oath* was too general, imprecise and pagan to accurately represent the core ideals of their increasingly scientific and socially influential discipline. Those in charge of professional mores saw the need for more explicitly Christian ethical rules of professional conduct if the balance between prestige and prosperity on the one hand and patient trust on the other, were to be maintained. Dr John Gregory (1725–73), Dr Benjamin Rush (1746–1813) and Dr Thomas Percival (1740–1804) made significant contributions to this project. This theme may have particular relevance in a fully privatised global health care system, given the prominent role Christian ideology is being allowed in various health policy decisions.

Gregory was a leader of medical professionalism in the 18th century. His *Lectures on the Duties and Qualifications of a Physician*, published in Edinburgh in 1772, developed a prototype ethical rule of medical truth-telling during a patient's terminal illness. Doctors still had so little to offer therapeutically that if the patient gave up hope, the case was almost certainly lost. Gregory protested that physicians in his day were too ready to brand a case as 'incurable' and call in the clergy, merely because the alternative was to suffer potentially financially disadvantageous blame for the final demise. Many patients were left to die without adequate pain relief, or other forms of palliative care. Gregory drew upon philosopher David Hume's writings on sympathy to stress the need, at such critical moments, for professional virtues of humanity, gentleness of manners and a compassionate heart.

Another leader of medical professionalism in this period was Benjamin Rush. Rush was a signatory to the *American Declaration of Independence*, which asserted as a 'self-evident truth' the proposition that 'all men are created equal' and are endowed with 'inalienable rights'. Rush's *On the Duties of Patients to their Physicians*, however, was not quite the mix of egalitarian medical humanism and natural law one might have hoped for from someone with this policy pedigree. 'The obedience of a patient to the prescriptions of his physician,' he wrote, 'should be prompt, strict and universal. He should never oppose his own inclinations nor judgement to the advice of his physician.'

Thomas Percival was an English physician who, in 1803, published a professionally influential work entitled *Medical Ethics, or a Code of Institutes and Precepts Adapted to the Professional Conduct of Physicians and Surgeons*. He was a close friend of Thomas Gisborne, an ecclesiastical writer concerned that medical professionalism might subvert common fellowship and Christian charity. Percival's *Code* held that a doctor's conscience was the 'only tribunal' and that his responsibility was to learn from his mistakes and make sure they did not recur. Percival based the rules of his *Medical Ethics* on actual cases considered by an advisory committee which assembled rules of conduct for use by hospitals in England and Scotland.

It became fashionable for American medical societies to append codes, derived from writings such as those of Gregory, Rush and Percival, to their constitutions. The first two chapters of Percival's book were used as the basis of Dr John Bell's influential *American Medical Association's Code of Ethics* in 1847. Bell, in an introduction to the 1847 Code, wrote:

> From the age of Hippocrates to the present time, the annals of every civilised people contain abundant evidences of the devotedness of medical men to the relief of their fellow creatures from pain and disease, regardless of the privation and danger, and not seldom obloquy, encountered in return; a sense of ethical obligation rising superior, in their minds, to considerations of personal advancement.[12]

Controversy surrounded publication of the 1847 *Code*. Many physicians publicised their deep regret about its drift from virtues of personal honour and etiquette to an emphasis on duties, responsibilities and rights.

In 1849, Worthington Hooker published a monograph entitled *Physician and the Patient, or a Practical View of the Mutual Duties, Relations and Interests of the Medical Profession and the Community.* This extensive interpretation of the American Medical Association's *Code* was probably the first substantial academic work on the role of ethical principles in regulation of the doctor–patient relationship. Hooker criticised the regulatory efforts of the medical profession to date, saying it had been more concerned with 'the science of patient-getting', to the neglect of the 'science of patient curing'.

When Jukes Styrap offered his Code of Medical Ethics to the British Medical Association in 1882 to use as the basis of an ethical code, the profession in that nation closed ranks, implying that such an action would infringe their guild-type conception of the regulatory tradition of medicine. Their supposed ideal was of the doctor as cultured gentleman, an unquestioned moral arbiter occupying a high social position.

Conceptions of the ideal core of professional virtues and principles were particularly unsympathetic and unhelpful to women patients at this time. Deviations from the male model of health, such as menstruation, childbirth and menopause, were regarded with suspicion as quasi-pathological conditions, and widespread professional gender discrimination inhibited attempts to more widely implement foundational principles such as that related to egalitarian treatment.

Christian theology was not directly referred to in the writings of Gregory, Rush or Percival. Indeed, some have questioned whether the foundational moral principles of the medical profession ever received an explicit theological justification, or grew from distinctly religious traditions at all. Yet their private morality confirms other anecdotal evidence that Christianity formed a major part of the background of the vocational view of Western medical practice. The role of Christian ideology in shaping medical professionalism today may be particularly seen in continuing concern about the role of doctors in euthanasia, abortions, or the use of embryonic stem cells in human research. Strangely, it appears now to play a less prominent role in issues of health care justice.

III. The medical profession and consolidation of the market state

In the late 19th century, the medical profession went through a period of self-regulatory nihilism, in which diagnostic and therapeutic practice was related more closely to proven scientific laws. Improved microscopy and the germ theory of disease, for example, overturned centuries-old clinical beliefs compounded from generations of haphazard observation, superstition, blind obedience to tradition and disease-mongering, which viewed infectious illness as being caused by such things as *miasmas*, evil west winds, witches or moral wrongdoing.

Public trust in and respect for doctors increasingly arose because of their ability to reliably cure some diseases through the mysteries of science. Cure, in other words, could now be projected as an objective and reproducible fact, separate from moral beliefs about it. This is what now justified an individual medical practitioner's behaving with the appropriate *gravitas* or appearance of virtue while his orders for rest cures were obeyed. It also supported the profession's fight to protect its state monopoly from anti-scientific interlopers such as practitioners of homeopathy. Yet the hope that never again would irrational ideology inhibit medical treatment may have been premature.

§*i. Professional leaders: Osler, Flexner and Florey*

One of the unquestioned leaders of the medical profession at the end
of the 19th century was Sir William Osler. Osler was Foundation
Professor of Medicine at the Johns Hopkins University Medical
School in Baltimore and author of the classic textbook *Principles and
Practice of Medicine* (1892). He emphasised the professional importance
of achieving excellence while deflecting praise, shouldering criticism,
and standing up for principle. He summarised the foundational ideal
physician–patient relation as involving *philotechnia* ('love of the art')
and *philanthropia* ('love of humanity'). In his famous Valedictory
Address at the University of Pennsylvania in 1889, Osler argued for
the professional primacy of the virtue of imperturbability, or what he
termed *aequanimitas*:

> Cultivate, then, gentlemen, such a judicious measure of
> obtuseness as will enable you to meet the exigencies of
> practice with firmness and courage, without, at the same time,
> hardening 'the human heart by which we live'.[13]

Osler stressed the importance of linking *aequanimitas* and compassion,
in order to discourage professional demeanour that exhibited a cold,
desperately imperturbable mask of reason and expert infallibility.
When linked with self-interested motives, however, he stated that
commitment to a professional virtue such as *aequanimitas* may
endanger patients in proportion with their vulnerability and need to
trust.

When Henry S. Pritchett hired Abraham Flexner in 1908 to
commence a study of medical education in the United States and
Canada for the Carnegie Foundation, he deliberately chose an
outsider to the profession. Flexner, a man of forthright opinion and
extensive experience as an educator in the humanities, had studied
at Cambridge, Massachusetts with the great American philosopher
Josiah Royce, whose central moral theory emphasised rational (not
fanatical) loyalty to a widening circle of selfless ideals that included
liberties and freedoms.

Flexner's investigations disclosed that many so-called medical
schools were little more than dubious and decrepit commercial

enterprises run by cliques of avaricious local practitioners loosely connected with a hospital. His widely respected and studied report *Medical Education in the United States and Canada*, published by the Carnegie Foundation in 1910, ushered in a raft of medical reforms in North American medical education.

In 1912, Flexner was commissioned to make a similar survey of European medical schools. Though impressed by English students' access to good clinical teaching, Flexner particularly appreciated the German professors, who combined training students with advancing scientific knowledge. In language tacitly supporting eugenics, he praised German medical practitioners, who were struggling for 'economic rehabilitation'. These doctors and social reformers eager to improve 'moral and hygienic' conditions were now united, he noted, in an effort to place more 'intelligent' legislation on the statute books.

The general principles Flexner enunciated in his landmark reports have since profoundly influenced discussions of medical school curriculum reform and are likely to remain relevant even in an era of fully privatised global health care. The essential elements of the Flexnerian program included the following, all of which are relevant to our consideration of medical professionalism:

1. Emphasis on critical analysis, problem-solving and intellectual inquiry;
2. Organic relationships between medical schools and their communities;
3. Medical curricula that confront public health issues, including prevention of illness;
4. Educational opportunities in medical schools for children from all socio-economic and cultural backgrounds, but not to the detriment of quality;
5. Full-time appointments to medical schools, with such clinicians barred from all but charity work in the interests of teaching; and
6. Resistance to commercialisation. (According to Flexner, crushing the commercial impulse in medicine was a moral imperative.)

Yet in all his reports Flexner failed to recommend changes in medical ethics education. For example, he did not mention that since 1902, Charles P. Emerson, at Johns Hopkins, had encouraged medical students to work closely with the Charity Organisation Society of Baltimore. Emerson assigned each student one or two poor families to get to know over months or years. The object was not to study their diseases, but to learn 'how the poor man lives, works and thinks; what his problems are; what burdens he must bear'. When, in 1911, Emerson became Dean of the Indiana University Medical School, he similarly introduced a compulsory course in which students visited factories, as well as public welfare and philanthropic agencies. During the same period, at the Massachusetts General Hospital, Dr Richard Cabot also championed a 'democratic' doctor–patient relationship where the doctor was no longer a 'little tin God', but a person for whom conscience mattered, who listened to the patient's soul, empathetically overcoming racial and cultural prejudices, or conflicting loyalties to the state.

Some leaders of the medical profession championed global public goods even at this point. Howard Florey, an Australian, while Chair of the Dunn School of Pathology at Oxford University, assembled the team that isolated and developed the revolutionary antibiotic penicillin. Florey (backed by senior members of the UK medical establishment) refused to patent the invention. Florey stated: 'The people have paid for this work and they should have the benefits made freely available to them.' It is problematic what patent claim Florey's group would have been able to sustain, given the variety of strains and manufacturing processes that followed. Nonetheless, Florey's stand against commercialisation of medical research with immediate, widespread public health significance remains an important beacon in the history of medical professionalism.

§ii. Nuremberg: Medical professionalism and obedience

Flexner's reports failed to generally consider not only the ethical side of medical education, but also the possible deleterious influence upon medical professionalism of legislation in many North American States and Germany that implemented eugenics policies. Such policies often involved efforts to metaphorically 'weed Mendel's garden', to minimise the transmission of 'deleterious' genes amongst a governed population. Relevant 'moral hygiene' techniques which were becoming increasingly prominent in Flexner's day included laws requiring physicians to participate in compulsory sterilisations and involuntary euthanasia of purportedly genetically abnormal persons, as well as rules that banned interracial marriage, restricted immigration and encouraged the abortion of any fetus likely (because of one or both of its parents' genetic status) to have 'undesirable' physical characteristics.

From 1934, a doctor sat on each one of Germany's 181 Genetic Health Courts. By 1942, half of all that nation's doctors had voluntarily joined the Nazi Party, many (as is so often the case under totalitarian or liberty-restricting regimes) simply as a matter of survival for themselves and their families. Others, however, appeared to freely and openly endorse state propaganda viewing some patients as 'inferior' or 'non-human'.

On 20 August 1947, several decades after Flexner's reports had ignored the problem, an Allied military tribunal sentenced four leading German doctors to death by hanging. Their proven crimes included non-consensual, brutal experimentation upon patients, as well as sterilisation and active, non-voluntary euthanasia. As Brigadier General Telford Taylor concluded his opening statement for the prosecution, he accused those leaders of the German medical profession then in the dock of betraying both the foundational virtues and the ethical principles of their profession. This was, he said, no mere murder trial, because the defendants were physicians who had sworn to 'do no harm' and to abide by the principles of the *Hippocratic Oath*.

The three judges of the 1947 Nuremberg tribunal investigating the conduct of experiments by Nazi doctors were extremely concerned to find these leaders of the German medical profession championing obedience to law ahead of the interests of their patients. In response, they enunciated the *Nuremberg Code*, a statement of ten moral and legal prerequisites for the use of human beings in experimentation. Central to it was the requirement of free consent before medical experimentation. The *Nuremberg Code* pushed the ethical principle of respect for patient autonomy to the forefront of regulatory thinking about medical professionalism.

Some viewed the *Nuremberg Code* as a type of historical accident, triggered by the barbarities of war. Others, however, have regarded it as espousing a natural law obligation on doctors to loyally champion the welfare or good of patients, even if that means disobeying state policies and legislation. In any event, the circumstances promoting its revolutionary idealism were hardly a triumph of leadership in medical professionalism. In fact, the *Nuremberg Code* was never adopted in its entirety by any major medical association. Neither was it formally adopted by international convention or treaty, though its primary consent principle has been incorporated into international law in Article 7 of the United Nations' *International Covenant on Civil and Political Rights* (*ICCPR*).

§iii. Universal health care v privatisation and consumer choice

The *Nuremberg Code* was a factor in the World Medical Association's postwar (1948) redrafting of the *Hippocratic Oath* as the *Geneva Declaration*. In idealistic language that echoes that of the *Universal Declaration of Human Rights,* the *Geneva Declaration* reaffirmed that doctors had consecrated their lives to the service of humanity, and that it was expected they would practise with 'conscience' and 'dignity'. The 'health' of their patient was to be their *first* consideration despite any considerations of religion, nationality, race, party politics or social standing. *Even under threat*, they were not to use their medical knowledge contrary to the 'laws of humanity' (emphasis added). Similarly, the World Medical Association's 1949 *International Code of Medical Ethics* idealistically declared that a doctor owed to his or her patient 'complete loyalty and all the resources of his [or her] science'.

The *Geneva Declaration*'s requirement for medical practice with 'conscience and dignity' emerged contemporaneously with the vision expressed by the philosopher Jacques Maritain while assisting with the drafting of the preamble of the United Nations' *Universal Declaration of Human Rights*. This recognised that the 'inherent dignity and the equal and inalienable rights of all members of the human family' were the 'foundation of freedom, justice and peace in the world'. Maritain hoped formal international commitment to these sentiments would sustain a moral common denominator in global governance systems that was conducive to world peace.

This tripartite *International Bill of Patient Human Rights* was established to protect patients from adverse influences by the state on medical professionalism. It also contained idealistic principles that some leaders of health policy (Ben Chifley, Tommy Douglas and Nye Bevan in Australia, Canada and the United Kingdom respectively) drew upon, in part to honour the sacrifice of the fallen, to forge systems of universal (taxpayer-funded) access to health care and/or essential medicines. These health policy reformers were not doctors, but they challenged the medical profession to live up to its ideals. Their universalist health schemes initially produced antagonistic responses because of the supposed threat of 'socialised' medicine to professional incomes. In time, however, majority opinion amongst the medical profession swung behind the egalitarian idealism inherent in such public health legislation.

Yet in many nations, the Faustian bargain by which doctors gained a lucrative monopoly from the state continued after World War II to encourage doctors to acquiesce in becoming agents of state policies that opposed *Geneva Declaration* principles such as those requiring egalitarian treatment. Under apartheid rule in South Africa, for example, professional regulatory bodies determined that racial discrimination in the provision of health care by a physician did not constitute professional misconduct and that an equalisation fund to achieve salary parity for black doctors should be rejected. In communist East Germany, after military shootings of people attempting to escape over the Berlin Wall between 1961 and 1989, doctors falsified medical records and death certificates to disguise the cause of death and acquiesced in delays of treatment.

From the 1950s until the 1980s, the medical profession enjoyed significant social prestige throughout the world. This social capital had been constructed through the profession's commitment to the advance of scientific diagnostics and therapeutics, as well as by dedicated clinical work by the leaders of the profession, over many preceding generations, often at great cost to their private lives. Notions of the physician as benign and wise moral arbiter were reflected during this period in mass media depictions such as TV's Marcus Welby and Dr Kildare.

But this social authority and prestige, by blinding doctors to criticism, may have produced unintended adverse impacts on patients. As one doctor put it: 'In 1945–50, the doctor was king or queen. It never occurred to a doctor to ask [a patient] for consent for anything.' At one extreme of such conduct was the famous and greatly revered East German surgeon Ferdinand Sauerbruch, who continued working in the late 1940s despite developing a neurological impairment that began to harm patients.[14] Another example was the doctor of whom it was said by a patient: 'I could never have built up a relationship of trust with this oncologist. Each of my visits was forty minutes long, and [he] never did a physical examination … There was much time spent listening to private and professional telephone calls, even arranging tennis at lunchtime.'[15]

The *Nuremberg Code*, the *Geneva Declaration* and the *International Code of Medical Ethics* eventually risked being regarded as largely symbolic public relations gestures. Education about medical professionalism was widely considered to be governed, in practice, by a hidden curriculum and, for some, a 'flexible' self-interested ethics that appeared to validate whatever could be 'got away with'.

In this period, which coincided with the decline of communism in Eastern Europe, health policy-makers came under the influence of an economic theory that valorised the role of the marketplace. Known in some circles as 'monetarism', it required a small measure of state fiscal control over markets through central banks maintaining a steady money supply (achieved by controlling supply of their sound investment securities). At the same time it demanded (in an ideology known as economic rationalism or market fundamentalism) a downscaling of bureaucracy, deregulation of industry and privatisation (selling) of public assets. This, the theory went, would allow private enterprise to achieve a natural balance between inflation, employment and production. Four broad categories of privatisation were involved:

1. putting state monopolies into competition with private or other public operators;
2. outsourcing, where the state paid private actors to provide public goods and services;
3. private financing in exchange for delegated management arrangements; and
4. transfers to private control of publicly owned assets.

The resultant privatisation policies appeared to be an extension of Adam Smith's notion that interaction in a perfectly competitive market by a myriad of appropriately self-interested consumers and investors expressing free will to maximise relative utility would create an invisible sovereign hand that mechanistically and rationally placed an appropriate money value on all policy choices. It was a theory with minimal interest in any wider social contract debate. Critics claimed that this ideology's application of the human right of 'liberty' to corporations, for example, was designed to create a *faux* democratic legitimacy around entrepreneurial capitalism.

Market fundamentalism was embraced by political leaders in the United States (President Ronald Reagan) and the United Kingdom (Prime Minister Margaret Thatcher), much as economist John Maynard Keynes' emphasis on government spending to cure recessions had been embraced by US President Franklin Delano Roosevelt in the 1930s. In the 1990s, it was linked with trade 'liberalisation' (which in this context means non-discrimination against foreign corporations) and embraced in what was known as the Washington Consensus, by the IMF (International Monetary Fund), the World Bank and the US Treasury.

Since monetarist ideology claimed that markets and prices were an expression of collective free will, it then followed, the theory's proponents argued, that many social problems (including poverty and lack of access to health services or essential medicines) could probably be traced back to some unnecessary government interference in the market process. Concerns that the side effects of market fundamentalism included greater unemployment, income inequalities and dangers to public health strengthened when the doctrine began to underpin the lending policies of the World Bank – and a series of World Trade Organization (WTO) trade agreements – which permitted trade sanctions (appealable only to an unelected panel of trade lawyers) against nations that refused to obey its dictates.

Such trade agreements appeared to move decision-making power away from the world's people and towards the executives of multinational corporations, their expert advisors and politicians who had become beholden to them (through campaign donations and promises of post-office employment, for example). Their apotheosis may be the failed Multilateral Agreement on Investment (MAI), negotiated in secret, without parliamentary oversight or consultation. The MAI would have allowed multinational corporations to sue domestic governments for implementing policies (such as environment protection, universal health care and access to medicines programs) that would have the 'equivalent effect' of being an 'indirect appropriation' on investment and so restrain its 'enjoyment'. It remains a triumph of business lobbying that political leaders were not only willing to implement such free market theories without requiring any careful testing of their predictions and assumptions, but also to so assimilate them that governments themselves (structures representing communities) would have become market states (institutions representing the joint interests of large corporations and oligarchies of politicians ideologically 'captured' by private interests).

Economic rationalism (or market fundamentalism), when applied to health policy, valorised ever-increasing production of private consumer goods, coupled with the policy rhetoric of 'consumer choice' and 'personal responsibility', despite the fact that worldwide, 20 million people were dying each year from starvation and the world had insufficient resources to support such a privileged lifestyle in every nation.

The policy did encourage flows of foreign investment and valuable efficiency reorganisations in health service delivery. But it also resulted in overall increases in national health expenditure, despite reductions in government (taxpayer) funding of – and policy support for – public hospitals, cost-effective medicines schemes, and public goods in general. Governments began to ration funding for public hospitals, or simply turn over their health care systems to private insurance schemes and private health management organisations with exorbitantly remunerated CEOs and assets whose worth eclipsed that of many small nations. Medicines savings accounts were introduced to Singapore in the late 1990s, for instance, to help consumers pay for privatised medicine, but they only caused increased out-of-pocket costs.[16]

One of the most notorious examples of market fundamentalism applied to a health system occurred when economists trained by the monetarist Milton Friedman (referred to as the 'Chicago Boys' in health policy circles) were invited to Chile, after the 1973 coup, by the military dictator General Augusto Pinochet. Their mission was to rigorously implement free market ideology. That nation's universal health coverage scheme was dismantled and private health insurers were allowed to compete for consumers in a deregulated market. Massive inequalities in mortality and morbidity soon resulted, recent democratic governments have striven to rectify them.

Critics in nations such as the United States,[17] China[18] and Australia[19] began to question whether policies encouraging private health insurance would sustain the social fabric and adequately alleviate the problems of access to health care for the disabled, as well as poor and rural populations. The United States, which has a highly privatised health care system, spends more on health care than any other nation, yet has life expectancies lower than many developing nations, and close to 50 million people without health insurance. Private health insurance costs are close to 30 per cent of average wages. The US privatised health care system is now widely rated as a fiscal and health outcomes disaster on most standard outcome measures.[20]

Since the mid-1990s, the United Kingdom, the Netherlands and Sweden, for reasons of both equity and fiscal restraint, have attempted (with varying degrees of success) to reverse many of the economic fundamentalist policies that were resulting in privatisation of their national health programs.[21]

This lack of political will to support public health care provided the backdrop to revelations – usually made by whistleblowers – about inadequate standards of care, fraud, and high adverse incident (medical error) rates in public hospitals. Paper-based adverse incident reporting or institutional accreditation systems seemed unable to consistently detect incompetence by senior clinicians; many such public interest disclosures only came to light after whistleblower-initiated inquiries were conducted by experts external to the institution concerned.

At present, universal public health systems based on taxpayer-funded equality of access still have great popular support. The majority of citizens in most developed nations appear to view higher tax rates as reasonable if the payback is greater security and peace of mind as they collectively age and are exposed to greater risk of illness. Yet despite this widespread popular support, many governments are still producing health policies that lack any consistent commitment to such public goods. Indeed, increasing numbers of political and industry allies are willing to assist the continuing push for the full privatisation of global health care. Why is this deeply unpopular policy agenda continuing, despite the high probability that it is deleterious for long-term public health? What will be the consequences for medical professionalism and society if it succeeds?

§iv. *Maintaining honour and noble traditions?*

The fact that physicians, around the world, are increasingly working in privatised health care systems means that they risk being subjected to contractual obligations that add a more complex and often problematic layer to traditional ethical norms designed to protect patients and their interests. Professional adherence to such contractual requirements may, for example, lead to doctors denying patients without appropriate private health insurance access to or continuation of treatment. It may inhibit physicians' capacity to complain on the patient's behalf about delays or denials of treatment, to order necessary procedures or tests even if they are expensive, or to advise whenever better quality care is known to exist elsewhere.

By the late 20th century, the knowledge base of medical professionalism, evidence-based medicine, had become increasingly influenced by corporate investment in and thus control over the funding, coordination and publication of randomised control trials (RCTs). The opinions of the most eminent and peer-revered doctors were frequently sought and influenced by corporate gifts – of biomaterials, discretionary funds, equipment, consultancy fees, honoraria for presentations, conference subsidies or hospitality, sponsorship of continuing medical education, advertising and lobbying. Particularly notable anecdotal instances of alleged increasing corporate influence over contemporary medical professionals included disputes over editorial independence at flagship medical journals.

In the age of the market state, direct-to-consumer advertising is likely to be increasingly promoted as an efficient means of providing valuable health care information to consumers. Yet it can promote prescriptions based on advertising hype rather than sound clinical judgment, and encourage people to believe that the pharmaceutical industry has a medicine not only for every disease they have, but also for many ailments they didn't even know they had ('disease-mongering'). Increasing numbers of patients rely for diagnosis more on the internet than on consultations with a doctor. Large numbers of patients visiting a doctor in developed nations have seen an alternative health care practitioner in the preceding year. This appears to particularly be the case for those suffering from cancer and HIV/AIDS, where the efficacy of conventional medical therapy remains low and the need for professional virtues such as empathy, compassion and loyalty is high.

Equally disturbing and worthy of investigation should be claims that health policy development is increasingly being removed from citizen control by means of sophisticated corporate lobbying of government officials, mass media advertising and the leverage obtained by linking industry health agendas with the threat of international trade sanctions. If, for example, WTO agreements facilitate the private ownership of global health care services and technologies, as they appear to do, their democratic mandate to fulfil such a strategy needs to be critically analysed. It is also important to examine whether, and with what authority, such arrangements could prevent future governments coming to power and reintroducing legislative schemes for free health care for all citizens and equitable access to essential medicines.

Physicians, as we've seen, have collectively grown in social stature since the mid-1600s, because of their profession's noble dedication to relieving suffering and its apparent quest for the scientific grail of diagnostic and therapeutic certainty, which would render human life free of disease. Such a discovery has occasionally been glimpsed, but never vouchsafed. After a massive worldwide effort, for example, clinical illness caused by the variola virus (smallpox) was declared eradicated by the WHO in 1980, and vaccination ceased. But this virus now threatens to return, via wildlife reservoirs, infected bodies interred in the permafrost, or possible terrorist access to government specimens held in the United States and Russia. Moves to strengthen the United Nations' *Biological Weapons Convention* have been frustrated by nations that are unwilling to allow access for foreign inspection teams and claim they require smallpox stocks for biosecurity purposes.

In fact, the global burden of disease continues to increase, through proliferation of poorly treated infectious diseases such as HIV/AIDS, tuberculosis and malaria. SARS, avian influenza, Ebola and other atypical, emergent, manipulated and drug-resistant viruses threaten pandemics.

Human suffering arises increasingly from air, water and marine pollution, famine, deforestation, ozone layer depletion, global warming and climate change, corruption, armed conflict, and trade in weapons. Yet it is only described as happening to 'patients' when it causes affected people to contact the health care system. In developed nations, primary care physicians deal increasingly with lifestyle diseases such as obesity, hypertension, diabetes, depression and drug addiction (upon which the bulk of pharmaceutical research and development is focused), and complaints of chronic pain, fatigue and psychosomatic disorders. Technologically advanced intensive care medicine is likely to increasingly assist recovery from critical illness and the dying process, but only in the developed world, and then only for patients who are wealthy and/or privately insured. Most primarily genetic-based diseases, though better diagnosed, still have no cure. Around the world, 50,000 people die each day from treatable medical conditions; 60 per cent of these are children under 5 years of age. Many more are permanently disabled or suffer unnecessarily from lack of access to basic health care. The extent to which increased corporate influence in health care is likely to either remedy or exacerbate such problems will be a major test of its democratic legitimacy.

Partly in response to these challenges, the 'Medical Professionalism Project' of the European Federation of Internal Medicine, the American College of Physicians, the American Society of Internal Medicine, the American Board of Internal Medicine, the Royal College of Physicians, King's Fund, and Picker Institute projects on medical professionalism, have attempted to place principles of social justice (particularly access to care and distribution of resources) within core professional responsibilities and develop a new global social contract between the health industry, professionals, government, managers and patient groups.

The next chapter considers how one might best set about creating the conceptual framework for a system of medical professional regulation that flows from a genuine commitment – on the part of industry, health policy-makers and other health professionals – to foundational professional and social virtues.

Chapter summary and cases for further discussion

• The history of medical professionalism shows an instructive tension between emphasis on conscience, virtues and egalitarian ideals, on the one hand, and the quest for profit and social influence on the other.

• Global health care policy has recently come under the influence of market fundamentalism, an ideology promoting an increased role for private corporations and a decreased role for independent government regulation.

• The 'market state' is a term referring to governments that have formed such a close policy bond with industry that, in many senses, their interests are mutually perceived as indistinguishable and superior to any countervailing community concerns.

• The traditional ideals and values of medical professionalism are now being challenged by the dominant influence of the corporate sector and the market state in global health care delivery.

• Calls have been made for a new social contract on medical professionalism and global health care, between government, industry, health professionals, managers and policy-makers.

Case study: Jamie's story

Jamie was a 60-year-old employed man who thought he had full health insurance cover. When he was diagnosed with a rare form of cancer, he discovered that his insurance company was not prepared to pay for an 'off-label' use of the drug he had been prescribed. Jamie found a consumer advocate via the internet, who contacted the drug's manufacturer. The advocate requested access for Jamie via a 'compassionate use' program. The employee of the drug manufacturer asked, 'Does this man own his house and some shares?' 'Yes. Why is that relevant?' asked the patient advocate. 'You know the saying,' said the company officer, 'that you put aside money for a rainy day? Well, it's raining now.' Should access to essential medicines become a matter of discretion (or pharmacophilanthropy) by officials in private corporations?

Case study: Norman's story

A medical student was in a cardiology clinic when a 71-year-old heavy smoker called Norman came in with a history of several massive anterior myocardial infarctions. Norman rarely took a bath and his language was coarse and impolite. He'd been told that angioplasty wasn't an option and had decided against taking the risk of bypass grafts. Norman was left with home oxygen, but the cost was way beyond his pension. To pay the rent of the concentrator, he and his wife had to use all the money they had coming from a small investment property that represented their life savings. The physician knew the cost would be reduced if the patient had severe arterial blood gas results, meaning a PaO2 below 55mmHg, which was way lower than this patient's. He was reluctant to falsify the record in this way, because he disliked the patient and saw him as someone who couldn't take responsibility for his own health. Do such institutional arrangements maximise respect for patients' human dignity and for the health care system itself?

2

MEDICAL PROFESSIONALISM AND 'INTEGRATED' REGULATION

I. Regulating medical professionalism in a new global social contract

§i. *Core elements of medical professionalism under the market state*

> And facing the wall most of the time he lay and in solitude
> suffered all the inexplicable agonies, and in solitude pondered
> always the same insoluble question: 'What is it? Can it be true
> that it is death?' And the inner voice answered: 'Yes, it is true'
> – 'Why these agonies?' And the voice answered, 'For no reason
> – they just are so.'
>
> Leo Tolstoy, *The Death of Ivan Ilyich*

Amongst the character traits traditionally listed as expected in a professional, to justify his or her strong facilitative and dispositional social power, is a commitment to community service that takes precedence over profit-making, throughout a career. Yet we have also observed that the development of medical professionalism has involved continuing tensions between state public health requirements, the desire for individual financial gain, religious ideology and humanitarian idealism. More recently, pressure on medical professionalism has come from market fundamentalist health policies that emphasise consumer individualisation of risk and responsibility, along with the value prioritisation of short-term budgetary efficiencies and corporate profits.

The preceding examination of the conceptual origins of medical professionalism has highlighted many other elements that may now be drawn upon in constructing a regulatory system best suited to the challenges posed by an increasingly privatised global health care system. Blueprinting such a regulatory system will be the task of this chapter. It will use the term 'regulatory' to include, amongst other techniques, rules and principles (or 'norms') of behaviour derived from private morality, from institutional medical ethics and bioethics, legislation, judge-made law and international human rights, particularly as enunciated in United Nations conventions.

The first consideration is whether or not this professional regulatory system should apply to doctors, other health professionals and health policy-makers. Clinical doctors in the era of the market state are indeed likely (at least initially) to maintain their monopoly as state-licensed providers of the highest quality health care. These 'gatekeeping' powers will continue to make doctors persons of particular interest to corporate actors in the health care environment. Such implicit leadership duties include being sole prescribers of the most efficacious pharmaceuticals and ultimate arbiters of disease legitimacy (that is, for purposes such as insurance, compensation, or access to expensive new investigations and treatments). It is doctors, for example, who will control 'consumer' access to expensive 'innovative' nano and biologic medicines, genetic tests, high-tech diagnostic investigations, surgery and artificial reproductive technologies.

Emphasis on the doctor–patient relationship as a conceptual pivot point for regulation of medical professionalism need not marginalise the place in the latter system of other health professionals, managers, industry representatives and policy-makers. Rights, duties and obligations will vary with proximity to that primary relationship, but retaining it as a central focus ensures system coordination towards outcomes congruent with any core egalitarian and humanitarian ideals that the preceding history has shown are more likely to be evoked and sustained in those whose work involves direct proximity to patient suffering. A traditional doctor–patient relationship may be said to commence with an express patient request via face-to-face interaction with a suitably qualified and otherwise professionally unoccupied doctor at that doctor's usual place and hours of work. In the modern era of health care managerialism and entrepreneurial government, this free consent model of the doctor–patient relationship has increasingly become anachronistic and largely fictional. Its popularised retention appears to now fulfil a similar role to the (increasingly false) belief (derived from traditional social contract theory) that most contemporary governments in developed nations arise from free elections, and represent the collective will of the people. Both are notions that sanction or legitimise power. They are predicated on the two sides having more or less equal levels of information, respect, understanding and freedom – where in fact each relationship (doctors with patients, and citizens with the state) is likely to become increasingly asymmetric and distorted in an age governed by corporate control over knowledge, policy and regulation.

Indeed, a major pressure on the pivotal role of doctor–patient relationships in professional regulation will be the fact that corporate strategists and lobbyists have facilitated the widespread designation of patients as 'consumers'. This title implicitly equates health care decisions with those involved in purchasing a house, car, food or clothes. These are inaccurate analogies, not only due to the uniquely powerful capacity of illness to create vulnerability and erode choice, but because purchasing decisions about medicines or surgical procedures are largely trusted, by those suffering illness, to be made on their behalf by doctors.

In any event, in the developed world, increasingly fewer initial interactions with the health care system begin with a patient's arrival at a doctor's rooms, or a hospital's Emergency Department, hoping for assessment by the duty staff (interns, residents and registrars) under the supervision of an 'on call' salaried specialist or visiting medical officer. Access at this point increasingly depends (in the absence of contrary specific legislation) on whether or not the patient has private health insurance with the appropriate coverage. In many nations, thousands of people die every year before they ever encounter what we would term (on any definition) a health care system. Other patients first encounter such an entity by arriving at medical facilities run by international non-government organisations as refugees after torture, civil war, 'ethnic cleansing', or suffering produced by diseases and conditions for which cheap, ready treatments should be available, such as malaria, tuberculosis, HIV/AIDS, or starvation. In a fully privatised global health care system, a growing proportion of interactions with the health care system is likely to be initiated by the demands of a third party, such as an insurer, the police, an employer, or public health official. It has even been proposed that a condition of access to health care services through public health insurance may be willingness to participate in research trials of new health technologies.[1] In the age of the market state, consumers may increasingly consider their primary health care relationship to actually be with the private hospital, or HMO (health management organisation), that has contracted the services of the doctor. It has been held, for example, that no legally enforceable doctor–patient relationship arose where a patient was given analgesia, examined in an Emergency Department and remained there for several hours before being informed that his lack of insurance disqualified him from admission.[2]

The doctor–patient relationship in its traditional form may be ended by mutual consent, expressly by the patient, or by the doctor; but in all cases only after reasonable notice has permitted the doctor opportunity to ensure continuity of care. A grey zone is the extent to which the doctor–patient relationship requires prompt disclosure of adverse events (for example, before hospital discharge) or extends into other duties such as follow-up referrals, prescriptions or investigations.[3]

The enduring regulatory importance of the doctor–patient relationship is likely to be that once it has begun, a myriad of moral, institutional ethical, common law, legislative and international human rights protections crystallise upon the consumer/patient. It is these normative obligations (examined in detail in subsequent chapters) that will most readily (but not exclusively) define the essence of responsibility and accountability of medical professionalism in the age of the market state.

In the age of the market state, some might consider that entry to the health care system (rather than entry to a doctor–patient relationship) should be the central focus of a regulatory system for health professionals and policy-makers. The health care system may be defined as including, as well as health care at various levels, public health policies and programs (often developed in cooperation with international organisations). Such policies involve health education, product safety and consumer protection, as well as sanitation, access to safe food and water, vaccination, quarantine, occupational health and safety and protection from environmental hazards. They also would incorporate medical research and development, health and life insurance, education of health workers at universities and technical colleges, construction of health facilities and the manufacture and distribution of health care products.[4]

In the era of the market state, health care systems are increasingly being influenced by management strategies and policies based on so-called rational choice theory and transactional cost analysis, both of which assume that most human behaviour is motivated by self-gain and that markets and prices are the best indicators of value.

Regulating professionalism in a fully privatised global health care system will intimately involve not only doctors, but also other health care professionals, industry representatives, managers and health policy-makers. Nurses, for example, are promoted by their professional organisations as patient advocates with increasingly powerful collective bargaining and strong conceptions of duty to patients. Policies are being developed and laws passed to permit nurses to take over traditional medical tasks such as prescribing, ordering diagnostic tests, referring patients to specialists and admitting and discharging them from hospital. In specific settings, such as Intensive Care, where each critically ill patient is typically assigned one nurse for any shift, he or she is, indeed, in a powerful position with regard to protecting patient interests. Nursing staffing levels are likely to remain a critical factor in bed availability and hence patient access to, or continuance of, diagnosis and treatment in any health care system.

Including industry representatives and even corporate managers and health policy-makers in a system of medical or health care professionalism is a natural outcome of their increasing influence over its structural components, values and outcomes. Such inclusion may require, however, significant broadening of the 'closed club' mentality associated with many professional traditions, and altered roles for professional standards supervisory bodies.

The second major threshold consideration concerns whether or not an emphasis on *prima facie* duties or rights should be a distinctive conceptual feature of this professional regulatory system. We have already discussed how under social contract theory such duties may usefully be viewed as an outcome of principles and (more specific) rules ideally made under conditions of social consensus. Some such possible duties readily correlate exactly with a specific rule; others will overlap with many. A few (such as rules against torture, genocide, child abuse and slavery) are likely to be considered absolute, with civilised societies requiring that they be obeyed under all conditions and without excuses.

Most, however, can readily be viewed as susceptible to being overturned by conflicting duties. The professional duties of a doctor to a patient (or health policy-maker and industry representative, to the class of patients) under such an analysis may be viewed as presupposing the possibility of an initial disinclination to their performance, which may be accentuated by selfish desires, or consistently resisted with the assistance of virtuous character traits. This understanding will be critical if a regulatory system is to ascribe responsibility to a health professional who fails to fulfil a professional duty.

The concept of duty is often viewed as the 'flip-side' of rights. Yet positing foundational rights in a professional regulatory system may involve supporting a less than utopian original position, one where trust and loyalty are expected to periodically be abused and not uniformly supported by the community or state, or powerful corporate lobby groups influencing the latter.

A better perspective, perhaps, is that human rights (both international and constitutional) can only exist within a community of rights-holders. Claiming a right can be viewed as a means of justifying one's action or inaction either morally or legally in the face of potential opposition. Most legal theorists now believe that rights claims involve networks of mutual recognition; they represent an abstract attribution that we make about the value of others' existence. Some natural law scholars claim that properly educated humans sense rights viscerally within their personality, just as they detect virtues, or conscience in response to injustice or suffering.

The third major initial consideration will be how to conceptually visualise our professional regulatory system. One influential model views regulation of any human activity as a layered pyramidal structure. Each layer represents a regulatory technique and the amount of space the layer occupies reflects its proportion of overall regulatory activity.[5] Most regulation of the professions, according to such a model, occurs at the base, as often relatively intangible, decentralised self-regulation. Rational incentive for compliance at this level is facilitated by the threat of escalation up the pyramidal structure through such areas as, in turn, enforced self-regulation (such as a warning letter, or a rebuke from a role model leading to repentance and penitence), command regulation by legal rules with discretionary punishment (civil and criminal damages and penalties, licence suspension and revocation) to, ultimately, command regulation by legal rules with non-discretionary punishment and a greater implicit threat of state-enforced physical violence upon breach.

Such a regulatory model appears legalistic, in that it places the 'big stick' – legal rules enforceable by the executive arm of the state (police and judicial system) – at the apex. The dominant role of such rules is backed by a philosophy of legal positivism. This holds that legal rules are conceptually different from moral principles and their certain and predictable enforcement by the state is legitimated by their creation, out of due and established process, by authoritative institutional sources. Yet excessive emphasis on legal rules in any regulatory system may reduce compliance by encouraging participants to become tactical players in complex strategies to avoid the 'letter' of the law.

Our task now is to consider how the factors and regulatory structures just mentioned can best be modified and combined in a functioning model of medical professional regulation in the era of the market state. Perhaps the most radical approach, consistent with the monetarist, *laissez-faire* free market economics that underpins corporate globalisation, is that government simply withdraws from regulation of medical professionalism altogether.

§ii. Conscience in the regulation of medical professionalism

In his story *The Fit*, Chekhov describes how three students, of medicine, arts and law respectively, romp out for a night of drinking in a Moscow brothel district. The first two come home merrily drunk and attend their lectures the following day. The law student, however, cannot dismiss from his mind the depravity of those who exploit young women in commercial sexuality. In bed next morning, as carts rattle the streets, he stares at one point on the wall:

> It was a dull pain, indefinite, vague; it was like anguish and the
> most acute fear and despair. He could not say where the pain
> was. It was in his breast, under the heart.

A doctor is summoned and inquires whether the patient's family had any peculiar diseases, or if the patient himself had suffered secret vices or blows to the head.

This section, like Chekhov's story above, explores the role of individual conscience in professionalism. It goes further and examines whether and how conscience should be a central element of any regulatory system designed for medical professionalism in the era of the market state. Conscience is often regarded as a non-physical component of identity, an active component of the soul. Despite widespread historical and personal intuitive acknowledgment, its existence, as a matter of either scientific proof or deduction by pure reason, remains contentious (as Chekhov is emphasising in *The Fit*).

Some see conscience as that vanishing point of present time and space where the eternal soul may be shaped, through bodily action, by the responsibility inherent in material choice. This, like the similar widespread belief that conscience, properly understood, has some connection to (or is an aspect of) a universal consciousness, is a natural law-type position. Those embracing such views might see a professional career as involving a protracted testing of their practical implications.

Nevertheless, whether one is a physicalist or a mind–body dualist, conscience can be accepted as something fundamental to human idealism, the most highly regarded professional careers, and most viable conceptions of regulation under a social contract. For the purposes of constructing a practical regulatory theory for medical professionalism, conscience may best be conceived as a love of integrity and socially valuable ideals that gradually aggregates core personal identity around principles consistently applied in the face of obstacles. For this reason, conscience, as will be discussed subsequently, is a frequent theme of canonical literature – literature crafted with exemplary skill, and aimed to inspire humanity's highest values, qualities and interests.

Witnessing another's suffering is an experience that should arouse, in health professionals, industry representatives and policy-makers, a strong urge in conscience to understand and alleviate it. Such mental responses are a necessary starting place for thinking about conscience in a professional regulatory system, particularly if that system is linked to an individual's desire for character development.

It could be argued, of course, that it is unnecessary, in constructing a professional regulatory system, to assume any inherent desire for character development (whatever that might be taken to mean) in those involved. Indeed, such an assumption might burden the efficiency of that system with subjectivity, a proliferation of vague intuitions and a plurality of often inconsistent values.

Conscientious objection is well established as an action of disobedience to a legal rule that a citizen (including a health professional) is prepared to make, and justify in public, by explicit reference to contrary considerations of principle. Implicit in this conscience-based disobedience is the claim that the law in question appears incongruent with important principles derived from civilised society's foundational virtues or values, as well as with that person's sense of integrity about the purpose of his or her life. It is, however, a public action not primarily designed to promote change in legal rules. This distinguishes conscientious objection from the equally well-respected democratic interventions of civil disobedience and non-violent protest.

Conscientious non-compliance is less well known as a mechanism supporting the role of conscience in regulatory systems. It similarly arises from a citizen's or professional's conclusion that incongruence exists between particular legal rules and important moral, ethical or international human rights principles. In this instance, however, the outcome is *private* disobedience of the laws. To be coherent with foundational social and professional virtues, an act of legal disobedience characterised as conscientious non-compliance must be altruistically motivated. The citizen (or professional) performing it also must be willing to ultimately accept responsibility and offer a public justification of his or her actions according to important moral, ethical or international human rights principles.

Conscientious non-compliance may become an important means of affirming central values of medical professionalism in an era when employment contracts, and the repeal or amendment of public interest disclosure legislation, severely limit the general release of information that is relevant to public safety but contrary to corporate interests. It could also be significant in situations where health professionals have the capacity to assist equity of access to health care by misrepresenting patient information concerning restrictive criteria.

A large part of our subsequent discussion will involve exploring the appropriate sources of the principles that a health professional, industry representative or policy-maker's conscience may use to calibrate legal rules in these instances, and their relationship with foundational social and professional virtues.

The following story is a well-known illustration of the regulatory importance of conscience in the health care setting. In the late 1990s an extremely influential public inquiry upheld claims by an anaesthetist at the Bristol Royal Infirmary in the United Kingdom that children had died as the result of incompetence displayed by senior paediatric cardiac surgeons. The inquiry was initiated not as the routine outcome of quality assurance process. It arose because the anaesthetist felt that his conscience would not allow him to be silent and that the actions of those surgeons (though technically legal) contravened other basic principles of morality, medical ethics and international human rights. He became a whistleblower, and as a result suffered professional ostracism and disapproval.

The Clinical Governance recommendations from the Bristol Inquiry attempted to reform professional regulation by requiring doctors to improve their communication with patients and maintain a drive to lifelong professional self-improvement, collaboration, patient advocacy and knowledge of safety limits. Will such a whistleblowing action, following conscience, be regarded as outside or inside the formal governance systems that influence many aspects of medical professionalism in a fully privatised global health care system? The respect it accords whistleblowers may emerge as one crucial objective test of the level of commitment to foundational virtues and principles that a regulatory system for medical professionalism promotes.

Giving a central place to respect for individual conscience may have other positive effects as well: it is likely to make a professional regulatory system more sustainable, by attracting ongoing community respect. This will be particularly true if it is clear that allowing space for individual conscience is no licence for selfish liberty, but a facilitation of the capacity for decision-makers to calibrate the (often corporate-influenced) rules and principles of that system against humanity's best aspirations and ideals.

§iii. Normative role of foundational social and professional virtues

The moral philosopher GE Moore influentially highlighted three meanings of the term 'ideal'. The first refers to the *best* state of things conceivable, the *Summum Bonum*, the Absolute Good. The second form of 'ideal' means an object that is good in itself, or intrinsically and unalterably meritorious. Third, 'ideal' can involve conceptions about the best state of things possible in the real world.[6] Moore pointed out that the crucial factor in evaluating whether an ideal represents 'good' is the strength (duration and intensity) of our intuitive and emotional response to it. Kant reconciled these conceptions of the ideal by proposing that the only thing in the world capable of being characterised as good without qualification is a good will.[7] Kant stated that a will was not to be considered good because of what it effects or accomplishes, or even its fitness for valuable ends, but because it consistently acts upon maxims worthy of being followed by all human beings.

Professional virtues such as justice, loyalty, courage, competence and compassion are foundational according to such views, because they both arise from and promote principles of conduct that are capable of universal application. They develop gradually in human individuals and groups out of sustained, emotive love of ideal behaviour towards patients and an aversion to those qualities that threaten it (such as injustice, incompetence or disloyalty to the relief of patient suffering).

The jurisprudential scholar John Rawls, in his influential *Theory of Justice*, attempted to design the conceptual foundations of an equitable regulatory system for democratic society. He did this by conceptually integrating certain basic rights with fundamental principles he claimed could be readily derived from the social virtue of justice. The basic idea was that by simple grammatical manoeuvring, a society's description of the way to be virtuously just could be placed in the imperative and become a prescription, or an 'ought' statement generating general principles and specific legal rules, such as those enunciated in the Constitution or legislation.

Rawls claimed to be heavily influenced in this approach by the works of both Aristotle and Kant. He did not mention, however, the growing body of international human rights law involved in the same task.[8] Included in Rawls' theory was much moral psychology and discussion of 'the good' in terms of individual, rational 'life narratives' and the enjoyment implicit in the progressively more complex exercise of innate and trained abilities. A practical outcome of Rawls' ideas about the normative importance of 'life narratives' is found in the *Philosophers' Brief* he wrote in conjunction with Ronald Dworkin, Robert Nozik and others to assist the US Supreme Court in a case about the legality of assisted suicide.[9]

These philosophers were commenting on cases brought to seek professional assistance with dying by five competent (not depressed) individuals in the final stages of terminal illness. Two patients had intractable pain from advanced cancer, another two were in the last stages of HIV/AIDS, and one suffered a constant sense of suffocation due to untreatable emphysema. The conclusion of the *Philosophers' Brief* was that the state should support, as a constitutional as well as general moral principle, the capacity of competent adults (acting upon enduring convictions that characterise their life narrative) to determine autonomously the time and manner of their own death.

The moral philosopher Alasdair C MacIntyre's *After Virtue*, first published in 1981, became a seminal work in the late 20th century revival of thinking about virtue in academic moral philosophy. In *After Virtue*, MacIntyre expressed pessimism about what is known as the 'Enlightenment Project'. This term is commonly used to describe the process in which a series of prominent Western philosophers, including Kant and most recently and contentiously Rawls, attempted to propound a rational, yet undeniably universal basis for moral, and ultimately legal, judgment. MacIntyre claimed that by the late 20th century, human beings in Western democracies no longer believed that individuals, or people collectively in societies, could march inexorably towards perfectibility, self-fulfilment or enlightenment based on rational thought. With no agreed end or *telos* to aim for, he claimed, attempting to resolve moral and ethical disagreements by reasoning from principles merely led to interminable debates (whose conclusions were marked by what looked like capriciousness and arbitrariness). It also resulted in appeals to the language of rights and duties made simply to influence policy-makers emotively.

MacIntyre's proposed solution in *After Virtue*, drawing on Aristotle's *Nicomachean Ethics*, focused on efforts to achieve character development through voluntary participation in community-oriented practices or roles. A major difficulty that MacIntyre skirted, not surprisingly, is that many community traditions actually promote prejudice, discrimination and inhumanity against those regarded as 'outsiders'.

Most recent work aimed at designing a regulatory system based on either promoting virtue or establishing virtues as the source of foundational ethical and legal principles takes the character and 'plan of life' of the decision-making agent as the necessary terminus of moral argument or policy debate.

Aristotle, who wrote seminal works of literary tragedy and moral philosophy, figures prominently, as we have seen, in systems of regulation based on hypothesised social virtues. This may be because

Aristotle's *Ethics*, which emphasises the tutelage of reason, is free (conveniently for this age, where moral pluralism and relativism habitually war with theological fanaticism) from religious associations. Aristotle's pre-eminence in such debates might be due additionally to the clarity of his thought, but it could also arise because of the culturally restrictive philosophic education of scholars working in this area, or their inability to break with limiting intellectual conventions. The teachings of Buddha, for example, would seem to create an equally valid point of reference for a discussion of contemporary individual, social and professional virtues.

According to Aristotle, when a person trains his or her reason to consistently search for the mean between extremes of consequence, or assertions of principle, this not only improves performance of functions, but also gradually develops leadership skills, character, moral dignity or *eudaimonia*. An extrapolation from this is that regulatory systems should look to the facts of what humans – health professionals, industry representatives and policy-makers in our case – need to 'flourish', that is, to achieve a life informed by fully developed potentialities. I will later discuss the implications for medical professionalism of actually incorporating this as a practical career goal; one that promotes the view that all life's occasions should be viewed as opportunities to develop virtue.

The moral philosopher Philippa Foot suggested that Aristotle's *arete* (Thomas Aquinas's *virtus*) comprise what she would call the four cardinal social and personal virtues (courage, temperance, wisdom and justice). These are 'correctives'. They arise from conscious and prolonged performance of duty at points where this is made difficult by temptation, or deficient motivation.[10] Kant made substantial attempts to integrate an understanding of both virtue and principle into his moral theory. 'The true strength of virtue,' he wrote, 'is a *tranquil mind* with a considered and firm resolution to put the law of virtue [principles and rules capable of universal application] into practice.'[11]

Some regulatory theorists might recommend that medical professionalism in the era of the market state be conceptually based on a single utilitarian goal, such as 'fair access to health care for all'. Yet Rawls, in his *Theory of Justice*, influentially expressed a dislike of regulatory theories based on such apparently communal (teleological) goals.[12] This is because their emphasis on striving to achieve a purported community good appeared to risk totalitarian abuse in the manner parodied by George Orwell's *Animal Farm* and critiqued by Hannah Arendt in *The Origins of Totalitarianism*. In such an oppressive society, individual rights derived from fundamental virtues and principles are regarded as secondary or dependent (tradeable or expendable), rather than primary (or inviolable). The idea that corporate profit-making may emerge as such as goal in the era of the market state is of some concern.

It seems important, then, that a regulatory system for medical professionalism in the era of the market state be founded on a particular professional virtue, much as 'justice' operates at the foundation of social systems. Medical professionalism may be in a unique position to overcome the problems associated with totalitarian communal goals, by positing a unique *telos* focused on individual, rather than communal welfare. The credentials of this proposed foundational professional virtue, loyalty to the relief of patient suffering, will be examined in the next section.

§iv. Importance of a unified professional virtue

Whether or not a regulatory system for medical professionalism in and beyond the era of the market state should be conceptually founded on one or many professional virtues is likely to be a major topic of debate. So too, of course, are permutations of the argument – often advanced by realists who pride themselves on having practical temperaments, extensive, bitter experience or shrewd perception – that despite all our best efforts, little genuine commitment to virtue is yet to be encountered in this world. A position denying any role for virtue in professional regulation is unlikely, however, because of its presumptively misanthropic lack of inspiration, to sustain morale, or any form of socially respected outcome.

Some may argue for equivalence: that a health professional, industry representative or policy-maker, for example, can't be expected to possess one virtue without possessing all. Others will claim that in a practical sense, all professional virtues are necessarily interconnected and equally valuable. The contemporary bioethicists Edmund Pellegrino and David Thomasma describe numerous virtues hovering, like angels, over any regulatory system of rules and rights concerning doctor and patient.[13] Yet Dr Samuel Johnson, that pre-eminent English champion of virtue, didn't agree. He viewed the virtue of *caritas* (caring with acted responsibility) as distinct from and superior to *compassion* (a psychological state that might never move to action).[14]

It was the American philosopher Josiah Royce, in 1908, who most comprehensively developed the thesis that a person's conscience, his or her motivation and sense of obligation to follow social and spiritual rules, could be centralised around a single virtue: a rational conception of loyalty.[15] Other influential scholars writing about justice or natural law (including Rawls) have drawn on Royce's work on loyalty. Royce saw his concept of loyalty, when stripped of its potentially dehumanising association with fanatical obedience (particularly in war or politics), as 'of great service as a means of clarifying and simplifying the tangled moral problems of our lives and of our age'. Royce viewed loyalty as a 'willing' (freely chosen), 'thoroughgoing' (comprehensive) and 'practical' (not fanatical) devotion to a cause. The cause required the restraint or submission of one's desires and impulses for personal advantage or pleasure, in order to serve a community outside the self.

Royce wrestled with the question of whether loyalty could be a good to the loyal individual (such as a doctor obedient to the corporate-influenced laws of a market state) despite an apparent lack of broader social benefit from that obedience. Royce's solution was to promote loyalty to the cause of promoting universal loyalty as the highest form of this coordinating virtue. This formulation, of course, has echoes of Kant's statement that the only categorical good is reverence for principles that can readily be willed to be a law for everyone. Royce claimed that a wrong or evil cause that demands loyalty (such as a government, in the interests of corporate profits, demanding obedience to pro-privatisation laws it knows will reduce the welfare of its citizens) is invariably characterised by the fact that it arbitrarily limits other, normally socially valuable, forms of loyalty.

The truly loyal person, stated Royce (for example, a doctor, CEO of an HMO, or Health Minister with an active professional conscience) is inspired to decisive action by a life plan in which he or she is loyal not only to self, family and social development, but also to the continued existence of an equally unique scheme of duties internationally, intergenerationally and even (in time, if extraterrestrial intelligent life is discovered) cosmologically. Royce's loyalty thus involved an expansion of sympathy, a reverence for, and extension of moral principle to, all life. Royce expressly linked loyalty with conscience, and stated that, as a guide, it could take us – much as Virgil took Dante, the personal notebook *Markings* guided reformist United Nation's Secretary General Dag Hammarskjöld, the music of JS Bach helped medical idealist Dr Albert Schweitzer, or love of wilderness led inspirational environmentalists John Muir, Aldo Leopold and Dr Bob Brown through the worst and best in nature – towards fulfilment of our world-affirming ethical potential.

Royce's 'loyalty to loyalty' as a supreme good, however, if placed at the core of a regulatory system for medical professionalism, could perpetuate the cycle of 'virtue is what the virtuous person seeks'. This might make it difficult for that regulatory system to provide firm (and if necessary enforceable) guidance for professional conduct. Given the difficulties of defining such a virtue, its central regulatory role might also promote a guild or closed shop mentality, rewarding behaviour that facilitated income and prestige protection amongst members of the profession. Making the foundational professional virtue loyalty to the relief of individual patient suffering may avoid such problems.

§v. Principlist bioethics and medical professionalism

In 1964 the World Medical Association, in the *Helsinki Declaration*, reaffirmed the principle that it was imperative for doctors to practise medical research with good conscience and a desire to safeguard the health of people. This communal duty, however, was not to take precedence over the wellbeing, privacy and dignity of the individual research subject. In 1975 the World Medical Association's *Declaration of Tokyo* on torture and other cruel, inhuman or degrading treatment or punishment reaffirmed a similar vision of medical professionalism:

> The doctor's fundamental role is to alleviate the distress of his or her fellow men, and no motive whether personal, collective or political shall prevail against this higher purpose.[16]

In the early 1970s, few medical schools anywhere in the world taught such principles of medical ethics in a formal, required course. After this time, however, bioethics began to develop, particularly in North America, as an academic discipline, a strong impetus being provided by liberal judicial decisions on significant health law issues. Examples included *Quinlan* on withdrawal of treatment,[17] *Canterbury v Spence* on informed consent[18] and *Roe v Wade* on reproductive freedom prior to fetal viability through a constitutional right to privacy.[19]

The 'four principles' (respect for patient autonomy, beneficence, non-maleficence and justice) were developed by Tom L Beauchamp and James F Childress (in *Principles of Biomedical Ethics*) during this period, to create a common language for the 'identification, analysis, and resolution of moral problems in biomedicine'. They claimed that these clusters of *prima facie* principles were derived from 'considered judgments in the common morality and medical tradition'. Beauchamp and Childress asserted that some such principles (beneficence and non-maleficence) had been consistently emphasised, and others (autonomy and justice) relatively neglected, in the history of medical professionalism. The 'four principles' were to be applied in particular biomedical contexts by weighing their specification as substantive or procedural rules, by coherence balancing, and by drawing on Rawls's concept of 'reflective equilibrium'. Corporate health care managers and state health policy-makers were not explicitly included in the system of professional ethics developed by these authors.

The four principles are likely to remain central to formal medical ethics education in, and beyond, the era of fully privatised global health care. Their sustained importance will probably be due to both their public relations role and the useful governance emphasis they bring through the cluster of principles known as *autonomy*. Autonomy requires respect for the deliberated self-rule of other people. It is linked to Kant's 'categorical imperative' to act on universally applicable maxims that regard all beings as capable of reason, as ends complete in themselves, not mere means to some other good. Such a conception of autonomy allows the deduction of specific rules of institutional medical ethics: upholding promises, maintaining confidentiality, truth-telling, keeping appointments and achieving the requisite competence in communicating information.

The strong influence wielded by health care executives and health policy-makers over individual clinical decisions in the era of the market state suggests that an attempt should be made to incorporate them within a functional and comprehensive system of modern medical ethics. If this occurs, then corporate health care managers may be less unaccountably able to manipulate an ethical principle such as 'respect for patient autonomy', for example, into a brand slogan promoting a 'consumer choice–consumer responsibility' model of health care. Such incorporation, as well as presenting a more realistic picture of the dominant actors in modern medical professionalism, may assist in preventing autonomy, kept constructively ambiguous, from becoming merely a convenient policy-lobbying principle for those attempting to reconstruct medicine as a lucrative service industry where access, quality, competition and funding are regulated, chiefly contractually and legislatively, by the market.

Attempts to explicitly link the historical background of beneficence and non-maleficence to the professional responsibilities of health care managers and policy-makers may also be important. Without such overt association, such fundamental principles of medical ethics may metamorphose into advertising campaign messages, for example, painting private health institutions as providing net medical benefit to patients with minimal harm. It will be even more important to similarly explicitly apply the ethical principle of justice to such corporate and governmental health care actors. This will help ensure that justice remains an important ideal for health care regulation in the market state: to ensure fair distribution of scarce resources (distributive justice), to respect patients' rights (rights-based justice) and to respect morally acceptable laws (legal justice).

Without such attempts to broaden the range of actors to which medical ethics is applicable, another great advantage for corporate health care managers in having medical ethics education reduced to teaching the four principles may be the relative ease with which this can be used to over-simplify any complex process of coherence reasoning in clinical decision-making and to minimise critical analysis of health policy.

'Principlism' was designed to be communicated through lectures or group discussions about relevant ethical theories (for instance, deontology or utilitarianism) and related principles and rules, as well as development of the cognitive skills necessary to apply them to complex clinical dilemmas. But its use of deductive logic appeals to the fascination with all things legal that many doctors have. Further, a simplistic form of principlism appears to have achieved an unsought prominence in the 'hidden' curriculum of medical professionalism, taught by (often cynical and disillusioned) practitioners in informal workplace interactions with students and junior colleagues.

The initial academic thrust of bioethics focused on developing and communicating theories and principles to intra-professionally preserve patient autonomy and privacy against state intrusions. Bioethics subsequently, however, became more concerned about issues such as the just macro and micro allocation of resources. This culminated in the social responsibility principle (Article 14.2) of the UNESCO *Universal Declaration on Bioethics and Human Rights*, which required states and corporate actors to facilitate access to both quality health care and essential medicines for all human beings.[20] By that date, most medical schools throughout the world included medical ethics, health law and to a lesser extent international human rights, as part of their curricula.

The four principles approach to medical ethics education has recently been subjected to considerable conceptual challenge.[21] Claims have been made that a doctor's capacity to parrot the principlist mantra gives little reassurance to patients that the doctor was not only physically at their side, but in conscience on their side, against the cost-constraining bureaucracy of an increasingly privatised health care system.

Instruction in the four principles seems insufficient, alone, to help doctors develop the skills associated with, for example, explaining to patients the ramifications of complex medical technology in relation to end-of-life decisions.[22] Many patients have become dissatisfied with the apparently immature bedside manner of academically bright and technologically competent junior doctors, for whom medical ethics appears to 'be' the four principles and to revolve around not careful deliberation in an informed conscience, but the signing and filing of pieces of paper in the clinical record. They grow perplexed that so many of the major structural decisions governing access to health care are made by managers and policy-makers with no explicit allegiance to, or accountability under, principles of medical ethics that have an established place in what may be termed the 'social contract'. Yet health care corporate executives and policy-makers, till now, have been regarded as possessing specialised skills – derived from training programs and structures for self and external regulation – so diverse that few appear to have even contemplated their incorporation into a single, unified system of health professional regulation.

Sociological studies of doctor–patient interactions have examined outcome measures such as patient recall of and compliance with medical instructions, level of return appointments kept, patient satisfaction, coping ability and treatment result. These consistently reveal a strong positive correlation between patient satisfaction and a doctor's perceived level of empathy and capacity and willingness to act competently and courageously upon it (rather than his or her technical knowledge of the four principles).[23] Similar conclusions have been found in studies of the placebo effect and informed consent.[24]

Those challenging principlism, or its extension to health care corporate executives and policy-makers, might hone in on its implicit bias in favour of Western individualism and self-determination. Suggestions that medical professionalism might be foundationally regulated upon such fundamental ethical principles are often now challenged with the claim that they are only fragments of a conceptual scheme that has lost the religious and social context which made it legitimate in a democratic society. There is far from a consensus that such principles were or should be derived from any ideal concept of medical professionalism. Indeed, some claim they were simply invented by the professional bodies (mostly without lay representation) that periodically enunciated them in codes of conduct. It is equally possible to allege that the drift of medicine towards a fully privatised model based on expensive technology is creating completely new ethical dilemmas, which bear little relation to the historical struggles of the profession to support the foundational virtues and principles of some ideal contract with society. It has even been proposed that medical ethics itself may need to become subsumed within international human rights to maintain its legitimacy.[25] The continuing synergy between principles of medical ethics, basic morality and international human rights, however, is likely to prove mutually supportive well beyond the era of the market state.

Finally, it should be noted that principles are generally regarded as becoming rules when they are expressed with greater detail and with more specificity. In a system of professional regulation, ethical principles supporting justice, beneficence or autonomy, for example, may give rise to ethical rules in codes of conduct, guidelines or protocols, about confidentiality, privacy, or the procedures supporting a fair complaints process. Health policy can appropriately be regarded as principles and rules established by governmental authority for the regulation of particular social issues.

§vi.   *Health law and corporate micro-regulation*

Undoubtedly one of the most cherished forms of scientific immortality is to be metaphorically pictured alongside people such as Robert Boyle, Isaac Newton and James Clerk Maxwell by having a physical law (perhaps an equation or functional relation) linked to one's name. We are used to thinking of legal rules as generally more proscriptive, and scientific laws as more descriptive of material tendencies and dispositions, rather than of actual behaviour. Yet the more that putative laws are made to describe the nuances of an actual event, the more they lose their explanatory force. The law strives to achieve predictability and consistency in governance by treating human beings as rational types; it rarely presumes to see any legal subjects as a prayed-to God may, with all their peculiarities of temperament, character, emotion and intellect.

Legal rules are deemed to have a greater relative certainty and predictability of application and a generally more precise and effective mechanism of state enforcement than individual moral, institutional ethical, or legal principles. They are not created to apply to a single instance, and are collectively known as the rule of law when judicially applied and enforced with formal (not necessarily distributive) justice. International human rights may both become general principles of law (under the recognition rule in article 38(1) of the *Statute of the International Court of Justice*) and be derived from them. Legal rules, properly created and administered, represent one of civilisation's fragile constraints on the use of force as the ultimate means for securing personal advantage.

'Legalism' is a term used here to describe a dominance, in attitudes towards medical professionalism and leadership, of rules accorded the allegedly authoritative status of 'law'. Somewhat ironically, clinical doctors and health system managers have become notoriously prominent in promoting this ethos, often whingeing about patients asserting legal rights while themselves increasingly surrendering their moral and ethical decision-making responsibilities to those expert in applying legal rules. Common reasons for such a legalistic professional attitude appear to involve a mixture of private employment contractual requirements, individual fascination with the social power of law and genuine fear of liability. It has parallels with the dominance that economic analysis appears to have in contemporary health care policy-making.

This is all to the public good, until one realises that in the age of the market state, many of the most important law-making processes, to varying extents, may be under greater corporate than democratic influence. Private actors, uncontrolled by systematic regulatory process, will have both the motivation and means to ensure that the law does not allow individual professional conscience (for instance through whistleblowing) too free a rein, either in the institutions they control, or in health care in general (via, for example, policies promoting public goods).

Legal positivism is an academic philosophy about legal rules that is likely to present marked advantages for the corporate managers of a fully privatised global health care system. Central to most of its formulations is the belief that what counts as law is fundamentally a matter of historical and social fact. According to legal positivism, if a law has been approved by due parliamentary processes, for example, it has to be treated as a law by citizens. This is held to be true regardless of the law's apparent incoherence with moral or professional ethical principles, or the extent to which its content has been altered by non-parliamentary lobbying processes, to reflect narrow industry interests rather than broader community ones.

The second pillar of legal positivism is the understanding that there is no necessary connection between definitions of the law and morality. Just as so-called economic rationalists see a free market as the democratically legitimate expression of social will, so do legal positivists view each institutionally valid enunciation of law as a legitimate expression of communal will. Legal positivists hold that whether or not a domestic law conforms to any community standard of morality (or canon of professional ethics) is technically irrelevant to its definition and enforcement by the executive powers (police and army) of the state. Descriptive legal positivism attempts to catalogue such legal rules as they exist; normative legal positivism theorises about what they should be. If people consider a law amoral or unethical, their obligation, according to legal positivists, is to engage in the protracted process of law reform, not to risk the consequences of denying the law's status as a law.

Gustav Radbruch was a legal scholar who, shortly after World War II, developed an influential opposing viewpoint. The Radbruch thesis held that a judge should consider a statute not to be a law where it was incompatible, to an intolerable degree, with basic principles of justice.[26] The Nazi doctors' trial resulted in a similar pronouncement for medical professionalism. The *Nuremberg Declaration* required that physicians (like those involved in cruel and degrading human experimentation for the Nazis) would never again have to obey laws of the state in priority to any conflicting ethical duty to relieve the suffering of patients. This support for conscientious disobedience residing in the heart of medical professionalism ran directly counter to the tenets of legal positivism. Many institutional health lawyers, policy-makers, corporate representatives and medical professionals, working in a globally fully privatised health care system, would undoubtedly sense the career advantages of supporting both the legal positivist and free market fundamentalist ideologies. Legal positivism holds that a responsible human (consumer) with nominal freedom of thought and action will wish to participate in electing a primary law-making authority (parliament) and thereafter obey all its duly created legal rules. Such a doctrine needs to more thoroughly address the role of mass media, industry campaign contributions, electoral fraud, and lobbying of elected politicians in the process of legislative development.

Modern apologists for legal positivism and market fundamentalism are likely to claim that it is a mistake to regard either as amoral philosophies, unconcerned with issues of bioethics or international human rights. Such norms infiltrate both systems, they might maintain, abruptly and avowedly through elections and policy responses to polls, or silently and piecemeal through a multiplicity of interpretations by a non-corrupt judiciary. Further, they could say, laws cannot be 'operationalised' without a moral ethical commitment to obedience on the part of actors such as the legal profession, bureaucratic administrators and the public. The regulatory 'big sticks' of revocation of state-sanctioned licence to practise, or criminal proceedings and possibly imprisonment, similarly would be viewed as largely symbolic threats applicable in only extreme instances of proven harm to public safety. Some legalists may even argue for the potential corporate advantages of legal rules governing most significant components of every doctor–patient interaction.

§vii. *Calibrating role of human rights*

We have already explored, particularly by discussing the work of physicians John Locke and Benjamin Rush, the conceptual connection that appears to have existed between the ideals and foundational virtues of medical professionalism and those of human rights. After World War II, the development of internationally institutionalised first-generation civil and political international human rights was seen by many as the start of a new global social contract. This section explores the role that international human rights should play in a system of medical professional regulation for the era of the market state.

Leaders of the medical profession have played influential roles in promoting a vision of human future based on respect for international human rights. In the throes of the Cold War, for example, US and Soviet doctors, led by Dr Bernard Lown (Professor Emeritus at the Harvard School of Public Health) and Dr Evgueni Chazov (Director of the USSR's National Cardiology Institute), conducted meticulous research on the health effects of nuclear war, based on data collected by Japanese colleagues at Hiroshima and Nagasaki. Their organisation, International Physicians for the Prevention of Nuclear War (IPPNW), promoted the message that nuclear war would be humanity's final epidemic: there would be no cure, and no meaningful medical response. In 1985, as recognition of its efforts to increase the pressure of public opinion against the proliferation of nuclear weapons, IPPNW was awarded the Nobel Peace Prize.

IPPNW lobbied incessantly for a nuclear test ban treaty and for an advisory opinion from the International Court of Justice (ICJ) on the legality of nuclear weapons, a ruling they hoped would play a major role in the delegitimisation of such devices in global civil society. The ICJ in this case was asked to rule that the use of nuclear weapons violated the inherent human right to life (article 6 of the *ICCPR*), the prohibition on genocide (article II of the *Genocide Convention* and article 35 para 3 of Additional Protocol I of 1977 to the *Geneva Conventions* of 1949), customary rules of international humanitarian law, various anti-nuclear treaties and the prohibition on the use of force (article 2 para 4 of the *Charter of the United Nations*). IPPNW continues to work towards an international convention that would prohibit and eliminate nuclear weapons.

International human rights law, strictly speaking, is a system of norms or rules that have found an institutional 'home' by satisfying the requirements in Article 38(1) of the *Statute of the International Court of Justice*. This distinguishes that system from more speculative, inchoate assertions of moral or natural rights, on the one hand, and justiciable rights set out in domestic constitutions on the other. International human rights law applied in the health area may promote state respect for individual patients, encourage state protection of patients from private (corporate) parties, and/or require fulfilment by states of certain basic public health entitlements. In theory, the international human rights regime is indivisible: all its components are equally important to the foundational principle of respect for human dignity.

In the United Kingdom, the *Human Rights Act 1998* (in force from 3 October 2000) required courts to engage in a form of coherence reasoning that calibrated legislation and regulations in that country against provisions in the European Convention on Human Rights (ECHR). Cases such as those involving the attempts by the husband of Mrs Diane Pretty (terminally ill at 43 years with motor neurone disease) to be legally permitted to assist her suicide display a fascinating jurisprudential interaction between the ECHR and the English House of Lords over norms such as the human right to life, the prohibition of torture and inhuman and degrading treatment, respect for private life and freedom of thought, consciousness and religion.[27]

Second-generation economic, social and cultural rights, requiring positive state action to be fulfilled, include the international human right to health. This is set out in the preamble to the *Constitution of the World Health Organization*, Article 25 of the *Universal Declaration of Human Rights*, and Article 12 of the United Nations' *International Covenant on Economic, Social and Cultural Rights* (*ICESCR*) (which creates legal obligations on ratified signatories, which include almost all states). It is also present in article 33 of the *American Declaration on the Rights and Duties of Man*, article 11 of the *European Social Charter* and article 16 of the *African Charter on Human and People's Rights*, as well as in many other international conventions and domestic constitutions.

The relationship between the international right to health and the regulation of medical professionalism is not clear-cut. The right to health, for example, might include human rights to taxpayer-funded emergency medical care, equitable access to health care, the basic preconditions of health (food, water, shelter and sanitation) or even the recognition that there is a baseline standard of health below which a state should not allow its citizens to fall.

The right to health in domestic constitutions has been invoked to make states provide basic medical care, including drugs and treatment policies for HIV/AIDS patients.[28] In the South African Constitution, for example, the right to health is expressed in these terms:

Health care, food, water and social security

27. (1) Everyone has the right to have access to –

    1. health care services, including reproductive health care;

    2. sufficient food and water; and

    3. social security, including, if they are unable to support themselves and their dependants, appropriate social assistance.

    (2) The state must take reasonable legislative and other measures, within its available resources, to achieve the progressive realisation of each of these rights.

    (3) No one may be refused emergency medical treatment.

In 2002, the South African Constitutional Court unanimously found that the government's HIV/AIDS policy breached this section.[29] The court held that the policy of restricting the anti-HIV/AIDS drug nevirapine to 18 sites was unreasonably rigid and inflexible, and was denying babies of HIV-infected mothers outside those areas a potentially life-saving therapy. The court took note of the fact that the drug was apparently affordable, easy to administer and recommended by the WHO. The court's order for the government to expand its policy to facilitate greater availability of the medicine was tempered with the caveat that the government had the discretion to adapt the Court's order if equally appropriate or better methods of preventing mother-to-child transmission of HIV became available.

Monitoring mechanisms for the international right to health include reports prepared by United Nations commissions, such as those on Human Rights and the Status of Women, as well as the committee to which governments are required to send a report every five years dealing with their obligations under the *ICESCR*. The inadequacy of such a mechanism is highlighted by North Korea's fictitious or absent *ICESCR* reports, which have consistently failed to address that government's lack of response to famine, inadequate health services and other basic requirements of existence.[30]

The international human right to health, if it ever became associated with practical enforcement mechanisms (such as trade sanctions), would directly conflict with many of the existing aims, policies and processes of corporate globalisation. This is particularly true in relation to famine, third world debt and the arms trade, as well as the impact of globalisation on developing countries' capacity to implement programs for universal access to health care services and essential medicines.

One reason why international human rights may develop a calibrating role with regard to professional decisions about health law in and beyond the age of the market state concerns the potential for rapid global spread of infectious disease, such as HIV/AIDS, Severe Acute Respiratory Syndrome (SARS), or bioterrorism (through agents such as anthrax or smallpox, for example). Such threats are regarded as rendering many traditional barriers of state sovereignty irrelevant and necessitating international cooperation in the interests of public health; they also imply a need for vigilance in relation to the impact on individual human rights of resulting public health legislation.

International human rights law also has given medical professionals a means of calibrating certain UN Security Council decisions. When, for example, that body imposed economic sanctions severely affecting the medical care and health of people in Iraq and Cuba, those embargoes were opposed by leaders of medical professionalism on the grounds that they contravened established international human rights norms such as the right to health in the *ICESCR*.

When the International Criminal Court Statute was adopted in Rome on 17 July 1998 (it came into force on 1 July 2003), acts including those which could involve doctors either as perpetrators, forensic investigators or healers, were defined as crimes against humanity, genocide or war crimes.

Many leaders of medical professionalism have been instrumental in promoting a profusion of other international documents claiming to protect patient human rights. One example is the WHO 1994 *Declaration on the Promotion of Patient's Rights in Europe*, which seeks to 'reaffirm fundamental rights in health care'. Others are the World

Medical Assembly's 1963 *Twelve Principles of Provision of Health Care in any National Health Care System*, the 1981 *Declaration of Lisbon on the Rights of the Patient* and the Standing Committee of Doctors of the European Economic Community's (EEC's) 1967 *Declaration Concerning the Practice of Medicine Within the Community*. Also important was the Council of Europe's *Convention on Human Rights and Biomedicine*.

This brief survey has highlighted the importance of international human rights in calibrating the value of health laws within a practical system of professional regulation in and beyond the era of the market state. Another important potential role for international human rights in such a system is to balance pressures upon health policy arising from international trade agreements.

§viii. International trade agreements: The corporate voice in public health

The idea that major structural and attitudinal changes relevant to medical professionalism are being orchestrated, often deleteriously in terms of relieving the global and domestic burden of illness, by the business plans of influential corporate actors enforced through the dispute settlement mechanisms of multilateral and bilateral trade agreements, is no longer a controversial thesis.[31] This fundamental feature of market state health policy confronts traditional and widely held assumptions about parliamentary sovereignty and the rule of law, as well as the role in professional regulation of medical ethics and international human rights.

The two multilateral trade agreements particularly important in this context are the WTO's *General Agreement on Trade in Services* (GATS) and *Agreement on Trade Related Intellectual Property Rights* (TRIPs). Bilateral trade agreements with significant health policy components include the *Australia–United States Free Trade Agreement* (AUSFTA) and the *South Korea–US Free Trade Agreement* (KORUSFTA).

The WTO TRIPs agreement creates primary obligations on signatory member states, enforceable by threat of trade sanctions, to pass legislation for expanded minimum levels of patent monopoly protection over intellectual property (20 years under article 28) for products and processes (particularly pharmaceuticals) that, under article 27, are new, involve an 'inventive step' and are 'capable of industrial application'.

The driving force behind the TRIPs agreement was an Intellectual Property Committee, whose members were key executives from the multinational corporations Bristol Myers, Dupont, General Electric, Hewlett Packard, IBM, Johnson and Johnson, Merck, Monsanto, Pfizer, Rockwell and Warner.[32] TRIPs was designed to ensure that intellectual property in areas such as pharmaceuticals remained a private, monopolistic rent-making right (in reality, of well-resourced transnational corporations), not something generated, for example, in the intellectual commons for collective good by taxpayer-funded university medical schools, or the profession.

TRIPs arguably permits the modern-day metaphoric corporate barons of medically relevant knowledge to shape the direction of research, as well as government expenditure in areas such as pharmaceuticals, and through them, the structure and ethos of medical professionalism. The countervailing argument is that strong intellectual property protection, by attracting investment and encouraging technological innovation, will enhance economic growth and so is in the interest of all countries.

Minor concessions to TRIPs obligations were allowed, after intense lobbying by developing nations. These permitted limited exceptions to pharmaceutical patents (article 30) and compulsory licensing for medicines production (after payment of reasonable compensation) for public health reasons (article 31), as well as staggered implementation dates.[33] Developed countries promised to grant access to their agricultural markets to developing nations in return for the latters' agreement to TRIPs. Failure to deliver on this promise has led to a degree of cynicism about and stalling of the WTO process in developing nations.

Despite frequently threatening to use compulsory licences (for example during the anthrax bioterrorist crisis), the United States has, since TRIPs was signed, been actively lobbying to restrict other nations' access to even these modest flexibilities in the application of intellectual monopoly protections. The United States has also been using bilateral trade agreements such as the AUSFTA and KORUSFTA to attempt to circumvent the social justice clarification of intellectual property rights over pharmaceuticals enunciated in the *Doha Declaration on TRIPs and Public Health*. This WTO instrument says that 'trade agreements should be interpreted and implemented to protect public health and promote universal access to medicines'.[34] US trade negotiators, for example, routinely appear to ignore section 2101(b)(4)(C) of the *Trade Promotion Authority Act* 2002 (US), which requires them to ensure that their trade agreements uphold the *Doha Declaration*.

GATS is a WTO agreement setting rules, backed by trade sanctions, for the 'liberalisation' or 'free market access' of global trade in services by private transnational corporations. It can justifiably be viewed as an enforcement mechanism on a global scale for policies derived from the ideology of free market economic rationalism. The influential US Coalition of Service Industries (CSI) has stated that its GATS objectives are to obtain, through successive rounds of negotiations and Mutual Recognition Agreements (MRAs):

i. globally transparent licensing of health care professionals and facilities;

ii. market access and national treatment commitments for all health care services cross border;

iii. majority foreign ownership of health care facilities; and

iv. inclusion of health care in WTO government procurement disciplines.[35]

The process of health care privatisation envisaged by such trade agreements is often promoted as attracting foreign investment in infrastructure, improving service quality, increasing efficiency and facilitating innovation through competition. Yet in reality such benefits only flow to communities with administrations that have considerable experience in handling corporate lobbyists and retaining strong market levers, including anti-monopoly, as well as consumer and environment protection, laws.

The negative case, however, about what happens most often after a bout of health care privatisation does not suggest that the corporate representatives and health policy-makers involved routinely have clear commitments to either medical ethics or international human rights. Efficiency tends to be achieved by staff lay-offs, market power congests and congeals, cartelism, tax-evasion, corruption and fraud proliferate, and regulators are influenced by institutional cost-recovery and 'revolving-door' private–public employment schemes. Private companies, 'cherry picking' their investments for profitability, create great divisions in access to services between rich and poor. Social inequality is also promoted by the removal of public utility cross-subsidies. Contracts are leveraged to give corporate investors a guaranteed rate of return and protections from fluctuations in local currency and demand. Governments often end up subsidising the socially selective benefits of private health insurance, rather than universal health care, and the community suffers from loss of democratic control over its social infrastructure.

Through successive rounds of WTO negotiations (led by representatives of wealthy industrialised nations only, and characterised by secretive so-called green room caucus meetings), member nations are pressured to continually add to a growing list of services that will be opened up to trade, to the private sector. Negotiations on such specific commitments by countries are technically required to be conducted bilaterally (nation-to-nation) through a 'request–offer' process. These commitments are extremely difficult (that is, expensive) to remove once agreed to, as compensation must be paid to the corporate actors for any resultant financial losses. Clearly, any effective system of professional regulation in the era of the market state will need to effectively respond to the challenges from such trade agreements.

II. Practical issues for 'integrated' regulation of medical professionalism

§i. Big sticks, licensing or self-regulation?

It is time to consider how all these elements may best be brought together in a functioning professional regulatory system and to consider some key features of, and objections to, such a construction.

Modern regulatory theory supports the proposition that for an area such as medical professionalism, the most valuable control mechanisms should not exclusively focus on legal rules, however these are defined. Educative techniques involving mentoring, role-modelling and use of medical humanities, as well as instruction in health-related human rights, are useful adjuncts. In practical terms, decentralised, non-legal, grass-roots controls include a mixture of informal techniques that can either enhance esteem and pride in the excellence and community value of performance or seek to undermine confidence and job satisfaction (by shunning, vilification, humiliation, ridicule, for instance). Also relevant are membership-filtering screens (professional admission standards) and all the other factors that contribute to or disturb workplace harmony, such as availability of leave, staffing levels, office space and outlook. In the corporate world, such control mechanisms could include self-regulatory guidelines, voluntary standards agreements and codes of conduct, as well as private market governance techniques such as multi-stakeholder initiatives – all of which are generally severed from legal enforcement mechanisms.

Corporate workplace protocols that deny virtue-promoting factors and are constructed simply to maximise profits will always suffer from obedience problems amongst an intelligent workforce. Like judicial decisions that fulfil a conservative ideological objective distinct from formal justice, they may erode staff and public trust, while merely displacing undesired activity spatially, temporally or substantively. Excessively complex statutory licensing or inspection regimes, or schemes requiring regulators to seek cost recovery from industry, likewise, may promote collusion between civil servants and corporate applicants. They readily lead to less rigorous and objective application of standards, as well as to risks to and dissatisfaction amongst consumers, citizens and shareholders. The crucial insight presented here is that any system of professional regulation (including one based on enforceable legal rules) is more likely to achieve consistent respect and compliance if it is constantly striving to achieve coherence with the hopes, ideals and conscience of those so governed.

It has previously been argued that the foundational professional virtue should be loyalty to the relief of patient suffering. Part of the reasoning for this was that patients, who are inherently vulnerable and susceptible to exploitation because of their suffering, should be entitled to expect such a virtue from their doctor, as a marker of the goodwill and values endorsed by that state-certified individual and profession.

I have put forward the possibility of conceptually clarifying this proposed foundational virtue by comparison with a well-articulated existing concept, such as Royce's unifying idea of loyalty to progressively more universal forms of loyalty. Such an approach could view virtues such as trustworthiness, competence, integrity, compassion and practical wisdom as special forms of the overarching professional virtue of loyalty to the relief of patient suffering. Relating regulatory principles back to such a unifying professional virtue would become a means of calibrating individual morality, bioethics and international human rights against norms of health law and related trade agreements that (in the latter instances) are more likely to be influenced by the goals of the market state. Testing the value of this hypothesis in conjunction with the main components of an 'integrated' system for medical professional regulation is the main task of the second half of this book.

§ii. *Coherence reasoning within 'integrated' regulation?*

Beauchamp and Childress asserted that their four principles of medical ethics could be 'balanced' through a process of 'coherence' reasoning, without the need to acknowledge any foundational social or professional virtues. Indeed, virtue, conscience, and instruction in the related theory and practice of whistleblowing, civil disobedience or conscientious non-compliance are largely absent from contemporary professional education, with its increasing emphasis on managerial control seeking to tame unpredictable, cost-inefficient governance methods. Pellegrino, on the other hand, has led the call for a single, coherent, virtue-based theory of the doctor–patient relationship precisely in order to sustain its place in the hearts and minds of society.[36]

In the 'integrated' professional regulatory system being proposed here, personal moral principles and those of medical ethics, law and international human rights form parts of an attitudinal 'community of principle' constructing the basic responsibilities of a very broad-based medical professionalism.

Coherence reasoning, when applied to such an extensive range of regulatory principles, utilises a valuable feature of casuistic processes: that where consensus cannot be reached about the value of imagined outcomes in a particular case, decisions can still be made on the basis of their relationship to a shared understanding of some relevant fundamental social or professional virtue. Such virtues in this context particularly include justice, human dignity and loyalty to the relief of patient suffering. Of assistance here will be technological enhancement of human memory, information processing and reasoning capacities, as well as improved scientific capabilty to detect and analyse virtue. This coherence process requires prior understanding of a wide range of principles, a capacity to accurately and rapidly acquire relevant factual information and an ability to tolerate ambiguity, as well as practical and moral dilemmas, long enough for reason and conscience to be convinced of the appropriate stance.

Coherence may be sought by regulatory participants across many jurisdictions. One idealistic aim is that it may ultimately converge upon a *droit commun de l'humanité,* shaping a more cosmopolitan, sustainable and responsible international civil society beyond the era of the market state.

Covert conscientious non-compliance, or whistleblowing, so reconceptualised, may be valued as quality assurance checks resulting from reasoning disclosing a presumptive incoherence in a health care institution's application of regulatory principles. Civil disobedience, similarly, may be respected as a non-violent (not interfering with another's civil and political human rights) act of *public* protest, asserting that legal rules (such as those produced by the market state) need to be changed to make them coherent with moral, or bioethical and/or international human rights principles fundamental to the life narratives of those protesting.

Clearly, corporate executives involved in health care may have the greatest initial difficulty with this decision-making process, which seeks prior equilibrium amongst such a wide range of socially respected principles. But overtly incorporating those people into such a regulatory system for health professionals is likely to enhance the sustainability of their organisations. Health policy-makers are likely to be familiar with such a process of coherence reasoning, but less comfortable with the type of regulatory scrutiny it may bring.

§iii. *Operationalising an 'integrated' regulatory system*

One mechanistic way a social contract might imagine this 'integrated' regulatory system for medical professionalism is as a pyramidal structure.[37] Superficially and most concretely, it could be divided into various horizontal segments, each representing one of the various regulatory components we've discussed. The amount of space occupied in the pyramid at each level may be conceived as proportional to the quantity of professional activity directly affected by that particular regulatory technique. Such ordering is inversely proportional to the strength of enforcement power the regulatory method can bring to bear.

Thus, at the base (where almost all daily professional activities are regulated) we have the unifying foundational professional virtue of loyalty to the relief of patient suffering. Society can expect that such a virtue, being an expected character trait of health professionals, will consistently be evident in, and improve the quality of, every aspect of each professional interaction. At this regulatory base we may also find overlapping social virtues such as justice and respect for human dignity. The next tiers, moving up the pyramid, would be general moral and ethical principles (such as respect for patient autonomy, and beneficence), then specific guidelines of medical ethics, clinical governance pathways, institutional protocols, international human rights norms, health law judicial decisions and legislation. The progression upwards characterises a technique as involving a smaller proportion of regulatory activity, but a stronger enforcement mechanism. The apex is contentious, but is likely, in the era of the market state, to be occupied by both readily enforceable constitutional rights and/or trade agreement provisions, all backed by strong sanctions.

Yet it is clear that this way of viewing regulation does not adequately describe what happens, for example, when the conscience of a health care whistleblower decides to rely on a principle of medical ethics (or international human rights) to disobey a law or an institutional guideline. Once such significant dissonance is perceived by a health professional, the solid regulatory 'pyramid' with its mechanistic, pinpoint 'rule' application, can better be viewed (by analogy to quantum physics) as an equally real, but probabilistic entity, in the sense that it fundamentally comprises waves of principle. The regulatory system's fundamental components, in other words, like the basic particles described by physicist Werner Heisenberg, become indeterminate but more multi-dimensional objects once conscience 'observes' them.[38]

To regard 'integrated' regulation of medical professionalism in this way, as both a solidly mechanistic, legally dominant structure and, at the same time, a probabilistic 'community of principle' emphasising conscience, like a gradually harmonising exercise of musical counterpoint, emphasises how that system is striving to achieve coherence between human ideals and reality.

§iv. *Relief of patient suffering, or shareholder profits, as the primary goal?*

The medical profession's approach to relief of patient suffering as a dominant regulatory principle has involved some notable inconsistencies. Until John Snow used chloroform on Queen Victoria for the birth of Prince Leopold in 1853, for example, even the *Lancet* demanded that anaesthesia and analgesia not be used to lessen the suffering of a 'perfectly ordinary' labour.

The 'integrated' professional regulatory structure presented here is primarily focused on the goal (or *telos*) of relief of individual patient suffering. Use of the word 'patient' (derived from the Latin *pati*, to suffer) emphasises this connection much more than does the term 'consumer'.

This focus on relieving individual suffering acts as a counterbalance to the profit focus of market fundamentalism. It also overcomes the problem that, though most (teleological) regulatory theories aimed at achieving communal goals have the regulatory advantage of providing clearly determined guides to action, they do so at the expense of individual human rights.

One problem with making relief of human suffering the foundational goal of medical professionalism, however, is that 'suffering' has a strongly subjective element that does not easily provide objective or generalisable data. To some extent, as Buddhists in particular emphasise, suffering is an inevitable feature of the human condition. Its coexistence with belief in a beneficent God, as the biblical *Book of Job* demonstrates, has been a theological mystery at the heart of civilisation. Human suffering, at least in mild and transient forms, is also an important means of experiencing the reality of existence and a useful check to pride and vainglory. The medical profession, as we've seen, has zealously resorted, throughout its history, to such arguments when unable to provide effective therapeutics. Yet suffering, despite such universal human experience, remains extremely difficult to define.

Careful analysis shows that pain is neither a necessary nor sufficient condition for human suffering. Suffering can involve any actual or threatened loss of self-control or intactness, a sense of vulnerability, powerlessness, an existentially damaging fragmentation of the self. One undoubtedly relevant feature of human suffering, however, is that it brings forth a call for assistance requiring specialised skills and knowledge. Its relief also necessitates from most patients an often reluctant revelation of intimate information, a compromise of dignity and a need to trust. Suffering, in the context of medical professional regulation, may be defined as whatever is capable, by reason of its severity and lack of self-remedy, of fundamentally threatening coherence in a patient's life narrative.

Restoration of good health, though often posited as the ideal aim of medical professionalism, is not given that position here. This is chiefly because it is, in my view, less likely to consistently arouse professional conscience in the manner required to inspire participants in such a broad-based regulatory system towards the development of social and professional virtues. When the primary utilitarian *telos* (the duty of loyalty to relief of patient suffering) is formulated prescriptively as the foundational regulatory principle of medical professionalism, it takes on the characteristics of a master principle, intelligibly relating complementary and interpretive principles – for example, those encouraging conciliation and communication rather than allocation of blame.

Relief of individual patient suffering is formulated here as a *prima facie*, rather than an absolute, duty. This is because suffering, as mentioned, may be so broadly defined, but also because this principle is not meant to provide any artificial reassurance of decisional certainty, through being used a trump or automatic override mechanism that dangerously truncates the otherwise often protracted and complex process of coherence reasoning. Further, clinical medicine, health technology research and development and health policy formulation and implementation must be practised with scarce social resources by health professionals, corporate executives and policy-makers subject to numerous competing demands, each with overlapping duties and rights. Finally, the patient should be entitled (according to respect for foundational social virtues such as justice and respect for human dignity) to indicate that some aspect of their life narrative is so critical to them (for instance their religious faith) that it be allowed to override the primary *telos*.

The following chapters will scrutinise key components of the 'integrated' professional regulatory structure presented here, particularly for their capacity to respond to challenges beyond the age of the market state.

Chapter summary and cases for further discussion

- In a regulatory system founded on social and professional virtues, a health professional, industry representative or policy-maker's response to patient suffering ought to consistently commence with a strong conviction of the need to care, coupled with coherence reasoning weighing a broad range of relevant professional principles.

- The 'integrated' professional regulatory structure presented here attempts to link the motivational advantages of democratic legitimacy and aspiration to develop virtue with the simplicity of ethical principlism, the predictability and certainty of legal positivism and the idealism of international human rights.

- This 'integrated' professional system, conceived as a pyramidal hierarchy, from virtue base to legal apex, involves regulatory techniques characterised by increasing rule specificity and state enforcement power, with progressively decreasing occasions of application.

- Such an 'integrated' regulatory structure for medical professionalism accepts boundaries between morality and law, the practical needs of state and society, or public and private interests, but seeks understanding at areas of overlap.

- In 'hard cases', when a law appears dissonant if calibrated against factually applicable norms of morality, bioethics and international human rights, this professional regulatory system may be more usefully perceived as a probabilistic structure of principles observed by conscience.

- Such an 'integrated' professional regulatory system, emphasising conscience and virtue, provides a long-lasting and powerful challenge to the inducements of financial and lifestyle advantages that might accrue from alternative models of medical professional regulation in the age of the market state.

- There are additional important aims here, involving each medical professional's character development and sustainable social reaffirmation of the positive values upon which the regulatory system is built.

Case study: Dr Scarlet's story

Dr Scarlet is an intern being trained under government subsidy in a private hospital. New regulations require Dr Scarlet to inform the Medical Board of what he thought, on reasonable grounds, was a colleague's professional conduct dangerous to public safety. He makes such a report. A week later, he is summonsed by his employer and asked to resign because he is undermining the professional reputation of one the hospital's senior specialists in a way that breached his employment contract. Tactically, how could Dr Scarlet have been true to his professional conscience in this situation yet kept his job? What principles and rules should he have been able to mention to make a public justification of his action?

Case study: Cheryl-Ann's story

A doctor in a rural emergency department examines an 18-month-old child called Cheryl-Ann, who has a middle ear infection. This child, from clinical examination, has no rash, but is irritable and vomiting, and has a temperature of 39.4°C. A hand under the occiput is able to flex the cervical spine till the chin touches the neck. The child now seems normal neurologically, but one of the parents casually mentions that Cheryl-Ann has been behaving in a way that is 'weird'. The doctor has to decide whether to prescribe antibiotics for suspected pneumococcal meningitis (in the absence of a cerebral CT scan and lumbar puncture). Should this decision also have to factor in the private insurance status of the parents, the agreements the hospital has made to only purchase a particular brand of antibiotic, the doctor's contractual obligation to follow clinical pathway guidelines shaping the most cost-efficient way to manage such a case, and the parents' consent to participate in a randomised clinical trial of an expensive new antibiotic their child may not otherwise get access to?

3

CORPORATE
INFLUENCE
ON
PROFESSIONAL
EDUCATION

I. How to cultivate a knowledge elite

This chapter road tests the system of 'integrated' professional regulation presented in the previous chapter, in the context of medical professional education. It examines how such a system might respond to challenges posed beyond the era of the market state.

§i. Corporate executives and policy-makers in health professional education

There is a famous painting by Anton F. Seligmann entitled *Theodor Billroth Operating*. It shows a surgeon, posed as a heroic figure, surrounded by tiers of (mostly) attentive students. Will this remain an appropriate image of leadership and medical professionalism in the post market state era? If not, what may become a more relevant symbolic representation of how health professionals, health industry representatives and health policy-makers should be instructed in the requisite values and principles underpinning their careers?

Well-publicised scandals involving institutional indifference and governance desuetude in the face of sustained incompetence by senior clinicians, or conflicts of interest compromising patient safety in health system management and policy-making, have undoubtedly been a factor in contemporary medical curricula paying greater attention to ensuring that students are acquainted with basic norms of bioethics, as well as international human rights, and their potential conflict with public health law. It is difficult to quantify what difference this changing educative emphasis has made to the commitment by health professionals to implement such norms routinely and consistently.

The hypothesis explored in this book is that innovative approaches to regulation of medical professionalism need to be created and examined in order to respond effectively to an increasingly globalised model of profit-driven health care. One related line of investigation concerns the benefit health policy-makers and corporate executives will gain from being incorporated into an 'integrated' regulatory system that encourages debate about their responsibilities in the context of the foundational virtues and principles that have emerged from traditions such as those of medical ethics and international human rights.

Many educators may be perplexed by the novelty of suggestions that they should run pre-registration postgraduate training courses that include health care industry representatives and policy-makers alongside health professionals. One response to their concerns would be that such involvement merely reflects, systematically and coherently, the influence of such professionals on contemporary health care delivery.

Testing this hypothesis will require curricula for professional education in health care to reflect both the idealistic aspects of medical ethics and international human rights plus the realities of market state health policy and corporate management. As well as learning to critically analyse the relevance of the professional traditions outlined in Chapter 1, for example, this expanded category of students should objectively examine such virtues and principles in association with the positive and negative features of corporate health care strategy and tactics.

Students could, for example, study the social and professional value of the efficiencies and quality improvement initiatives that characterise much private health technology production and health service provision. They could also analyse the democratic legitimacy of the enhanced corporate lobbying power over health policy that is derived from constructively ambiguous principles in trade agreements (and their associated links to threats of trade sanctions). Such 'lobbying' principles include 'transparency' (in reality, shading into selective protection of corporate commercial-in-confidence data while enhancing pressure on regulators), 'recognition of pharmaceutical innovation' (monopoly protection against cheaper but equally efficacious generic drugs), 'liberalisation of trade in hospital services' (removal of all regulatory barriers to private ownership of hospitals), 'dismantling of discriminatory price controls' (undermining pharmaceutical pricing systems that use expert evidence to reference new products against overall social benefit) and 'fast-tracking' safety and quality approval of new health technologies.[1] Students should consider the importance of such principles being thoroughly tested by democratic processes before they become drivers of health care policy.

Students also could be asked to critically examine the proven public health benefits and disadvantages of the profit-driven system of pharmaceutical research and development and the related global expansion of increased intellectual monopoly privileges. Does such a system promote health technology innovation, or reduce equity of access to essential medicines, as well as sustainability and responsibility in the global medicines industry, and how should these goals be reconciled?

The need for students to consider such issues is pressing. In 2004, for example, the WHO reported that between 1975 and 1999, the number of people worldwide who lacked access to essential medicines (316 active substances were mentioned on its 2003 list) had remained unchanged − at 1.7 billion. In only 52 of the 182 countries surveyed did over 95 per cent of the population have regular access to essential medicines. In low-income countries, 80 per cent of the population did not have such access, and experienced correspondingly low disability-adjusted life expectancy; the comparable figure in high-income countries was 0.3 per cent. In Cameroon, as a typical example, a course of pharmaceutical peptic ulcer treatment costs twice the monthly wage of a government employee.

Intellectual monopoly privileges, in my view, is a more accurate term than intellectual property rights for the range of issues involved in debates about the value of patents over new health technologies. It leads to questions about whether or not the potential ownership by corporations of patents over drugs, for example, should be regarded as a 'natural' form of property, like inherent rights to freedom of speech or against arbitrary detention. It is also an invitation to consider whether or not the social contact should continue to involve (as it did originally) granting a profitable temporary monopoly only as a *quid pro quo* for social distribution of knowledge.

Trainee health professionals, similarly, should be given the conceptual tools to rigorously evaluate, in terms of medical professionalism, such things as proposals to centralise research ethics committees, to arrange corporate-sympathetic appointments to key government research funding and supervision bodies, control funding of pharmaceutical regulators, or set agendas for medical education (by influencing the accreditation process or government funding to universities). Professional regulation could also be examined in relation to market state influence over public health areas such as quarantine, food labelling, blood fractionation, drug safety and marketing approval, medicine and health technology pricing and access to health care services.

§ii. *Jaded mentors, pressured workplaces and the 'hidden' curriculum*

A large component of tertiary instruction in medical professionalism still occurs through informal, traditional ward and bedside role-modelling. Symbolic induction, for doctors, into this apprenticeship model is often via 'white coat' ceremonies, or ward dress requirements. Their value is captured by the literary description of an elderly physician watching medical students rushing to a hospital through a cold winter wind off the Hudson River. These young colleagues had decided to wear their thin white coats, rather than more practical heavy jackets because, he mused, those coats alone seemed infused with such magic as might protect their youthful sense of immortality from the disease and suffering soon to be encountered.[2] Health system corporate executives and policy-makers, despite their increasingly dominant role in shaping clinical decisions, currently lack any overt association with such traditions and the values they symbolically represent. One hypothesis explored here is that addressing this issue as part of an 'integrated' system of professional regulation will make it easier for such influential persons to emphasise loyalty to the relief of patient suffering as their primary professional virtue with positive benefits for public and individual health.

Role-modelling represents a continuation of the 'glorious narrative' or 'inspiring example' method of virtue education – criticised by Socrates in *Meno* – which once bestowed an aura of almost religious sanctity on senior medical figures. It was, and still is, often marred by lack of prior instruction or supervision of the senior physicians involved, and by the cynical and jaundiced, anti-idealistic, 'hidden' curriculum some are likely to propound.

Role-modelling is only as valuable professionally and socially as the ethos into which it socialises students of medical professionalism. It may, for example, perpetuate discriminatory attitudes based on prejudices about socio-economic status, race, religion, politics and disability, all of which are opposed by the principles and rules of constitutional and international human rights. This problem will not be assisted by a continuing paucity of senior level female role models and mentors, not necessarily because women are less prone to prejudice (which is controversial), but because so many students of health professionalism are now women.

An overemphasis on role-modelling may also lead students, pressured by time and fearful of any revealed incompetence, to show a preference for docile and respectful patients, to misrepresent contentious information when presenting it to mentors, or to avoid critical analysis of mentor opinions. As an educational technique, it is unclear whether role-modelling will function as well in privatised health care environments, where clinicians are not adequately remunerated for teaching and are contractually obliged to prioritise their institution's profitability.

For an 'integrated' system of medical professional regulation to work efficiently, any lectures given, readings set and assessment tasks required on developing values of medical professionalism should be reinforced by the conduct of senior colleagues. If junior staff (and this might include trainee health system corporate executives and policy managers in structured observing roles) are adequately resourced, given safe working hour rosters and properly supervised, it is less likely that anti-professional (anti-service ethos) values will become a larger part of this 'hidden' curriculum via a form of institutional osmosis. This will be particularly true where senior staff are transparent in acknowledging research and employment ties with the corporate sector and students enter the workplace with a well-organised philosophy of professional values firmly integrated into their own life narrative.

Students of medical professionalism who are striving to become leaders and to reshape the 'hidden' curriculum should be able to critically analyse comments by senior clinicians that either denigrate the positive role of the private sector or corporations in global health care, on the one hand, or criticise the health-related activities of the United Nations and its specialised agencies, bioethics, or the regime of international human rights, on the other.[3]

Students of medicine, health management and health policy, under this 'integrated' regulatory system, should be taught together (for varying periods) to critically analyse both the advantages and disadvantages of free market economic fundamentalism as a philosophy underpinning global health care. They likewise should be provided with alternative role models through interactions with ethically endorsed or non-profit health care corporations, non-governmental organisations such as Médècins Sans Frontiéres (MSF) and Oxfam, other members of the international civil society, United Nations international human rights committees, and policy-makers from both private insurance and universalist health care systems.

II. Educating medical professionals for life in a market state

§i. *Developing conscience and critical analysis in medical education*

Education about medical professionalism and leadership under an 'integrated' regulatory system capable of moving beyond the era of the market state should begin with graduate selection based on not only academic results, but also interviews looking for virtuous traits; or, at least, nothing inimical in character to the subsequent development of professionalism and leadership (such as low tolerance for ambiguity, or inability to empathise). It should then proceed to encourage trainee clinicians, health managers and policy makers to consider their varying career associations with the fundamental virtues, principles and rules governing medical professionalism. A study of relevant canonical literature, moral philosophy and human rights jurisprudence may help hone the intuitive convictions, emotional responses and imaginative skills required.

It may also be useful for students to keep a reflective journal in which they try to mesh the moral principles organising their personal life narrative with crucial initial clinical experiences. For trainee clinicians (but also, as a more controversial innovation, for trainee health managers and policy-makers), these may include first actual experience of cadavers, patient death, cardiopulmonary resuscitation, physical examination, rectal, genital or breast examination, first invasive procedure and first proximity to a terminally ill patient or pregnant adolescent. Then comes calibration of these newly refined individual moral principles against those expressed in professional codes of ethics, guidelines, legal rules and human rights. Also relevant in this context may be institutionalisation of peer support and study groups, non-competitive examination structures and early, extensive exposure to patients at hospital, but also at patients' homes. Teaching should emphasise 'everyday' ethical problems that arise in the doctor–patient relationship, such as patient non-compliance, psychological distancing or a physician's inability to feel comfortable with crying, as well as similar issues in the management of staff and employees of health organisations. To become leaders of medical professionalism beyond the era of the market state, students must, as mentioned, also know the names and key principles of relevant legal cases and legislation, as well as relevant international human rights conventions and WTO agreements.

During this process, students should be protected from (and be encouraged to prevent others suffering) verbal abuse and humiliation, bullying, or poor ethical role-modelling. This applies particularly to students who suffer a physical handicap (such as mild cerebral palsy or any ailment that requires a wheelchair), or are discriminated against for cultural, racial or other reasons proscribed by international human rights instruments.

Medical students can gain practical understanding about the formation of legal rules and their relationship to ethical principles by acting as expert witnesses, plaintiffs and defendants with law students in mock health law trials held before actual judges in real court buildings. Such events could particularly facilitate an understanding of the 'integrated' professional regulatory system proposed here if they are set in a fictional country, towards the end of the age of the market state, where the organisation of global health care is part of a well-accepted renegotiated global social contract.

Increased promotion of patient safety through clinical governance quality assurance pathways, institutional strategies for prevention of systems error, as well as 'near-miss' incident monitoring through the use of portable computing technology, are other important educational strategies that may be conceptually derived from an 'integrated' regulatory model of medical professionalism.

Beyond the era of the market state, it will be routine for textbooks or courses on health law and bioethics, medical professionalism, corporate health care management and health policy-making to include a substantive human rights component. Students of medical professionalism will routinely visit police cells and prisons, witness interviews with torture, rape and domestic violence victims and hear presentations from doctors who have campaigned against such human rights violations. The hope is that encouraging students of medical professionalism (including health managers and policy-makers) to go through this process of integrating an increasingly sophisticated, detailed and comprehensive range of professional principles into their sense of self-worth will increase virtue in themselves, their profession and society.

§ii. Medical humanities' normative role

In the period beyond the era of the market state, the academic movement promoting the humanities (in particular, types of literary narratives) as having a strong professional educative function is likely to be integrated into mainstream regulatory theory and practice. The role of such literature will be viewed as not just remedying the way professions such as medicine and law exclude from institutional discourse the stories, unique spiritual and emotional interests, claims and voices, of those in minority or oppressed social groups. Its normative role will involve stimulating and refining conscience.

Humanities literature in professional education will aim to place the character and conscience of students at the heart of the professional regulatory system. In this it will bridge the schism between emphasising patients' corporate-instrumental value as consumers, on the one hand, and focusing on their vulnerability and intrinsic human dignity and participatory role as citizens, on the other.

The big danger, perhaps, is that this regulatory use of the humanities may fail to translate into practical clinical decisions and institutional change, and instead become either a romantically interesting leisure or public relations activity or a 'fluffy' burden in curricula under pressure to include subjects students perceive as more practical, such as anatomy, pharmacology, 'managing a business', 'investing for your future' and 'patenting your research'.

Literature, however, imaginatively promoting an active conscience amongst legal and health policy professionals, has been reported by educators to have a reasonable track record in encouraging empathy for those with marginalised social status, to permit 'moral reflection' and expose the use of legal language in the creation of social hierarchies. Studying Sophocles' *Antigone*, for example, may provide trainee health policy-makers with encouragement to incorporate into their conscience principled convictions about the foundational social virtue of justice.

Another pertinent example is Charles Reich's *The Sorcerer of Bolinas Reef*. This narrative opens with a law clerk describing a mentor relationship with Supreme Court justice Hugo Black. This judge allegedly 'had total faith in the fundamental principles of justice'. Many judges (such as those appointed by conservative politicians of the market state) shape the law by thinking primarily about abstract rules and regulations and then, often, their religious and political ideology. The first thing Justice Black, however, supposedly saw in a case was the human being involved – the human factors, a particular man or woman's hopes and suffering. If these had been adversely and unjustly affected by the law, this became the focus of all his compassion and indignation. The story concludes with the law clerk as a harassed lawyer in a private firm, ruing how, by helping to free a corrupt client on a technicality, he has tarnished the integrity of his own life narrative.

A purported canon of imaginative legal literature evoking professional conscience could include excerpts from Charles Dickens's *Bleak House*, Robert Bolt's *A Man for all Seasons*, Shakespeare's *Merchant of Venice*, Franz Kafka's *The Trial* and Atticus's closing argument in Harper Lee's *To Kill a Mockingbird*, emphasising the human right to equality. Recent candidates for this canon frequently mourn the loss of opportunities for heroism and nobility in contemporary, large-scale, corporatised law practices and businesses.

Users of imaginative, conscience-evoking literature in medical education claim its study develops a doctor's, health manager's or policy-maker's capacity to adopt a patient's perspective, to tolerate ambiguity, moral frailty and weakness, and to respect a wide variety of cultural, religious, spiritual, socio-economic and social backgrounds. It facilitates, such an argument runs, consensus-building or coherence reasoning in clinical decision-making.

Students of medical professionalism (be they trainee clinicians, health care corporate executives or policy-makers) may learn much of value from understanding how Dr Rieux, for example, struggles to balance his professional ethical obligations to relieve individual suffering, sometimes in opposition to quarantine laws, in a plague-ridden city (in Albert Camus' *La Peste* [*The Plague*]), or how Dr Franciscus tries to cope with his previously arrogant attitude to a now dead young patient in Richard Selzer's *Imelda*. They will similarly learn much from the reflections of Leo Tolstoy's dying magistrate in *The Death of Ivan Ilyich*, or Simone de Beauvoir's short story about her dying mother, *A Very Easy Death*. Margaret Edson's play *Wit* likewise imparts professionally valuable end-of-life understandings from the perspective of a female university professor, expert in the Holy Sonnets of John Donne, who is diagnosed and treated for terminal ovarian cancer. Dr Frederick Treves' tale of befriending a hideously deformed patient in *The Elephant Man* similarly seems crafted to awaken intuitive convictions about the importance of conceptually understanding foundational professional virtues, and then developing them in oneself through consistently acting under the impulse of conscience striving to apply a broad range of moral, bioethical and human rights principles in the face of obstacles.

Educators in medical professionalism might utilise, or create, works with messages relevant to the pressures likely to be exerted on professional conscience in a fully privatised health care system. Examples might be Graham Greene's *The Tenth Man*, which is about a patient in a phase one drug trial, or David Feldshuh's play *Miss Evers' Boys*, which describes the emotional tragedy of the nurse who convinces untreated black men to remain in the control arm of the Tuskegee Syphilis Experiment.

Of considerable relevance, in this context, might be George Orwell's *1984* and Aldous Huxley's *Brave New World*. These texts describe worlds where the state is seeking to impose a uniformity of life narrative. They focus on the struggles of individuals to acquire meaning through a privately moulded coherence between freely chosen relationships, virtues and principles. *1984* has the most acute prescience, describing a state apparatus controlling a populace through threat of perpetual war, manipulation of language and thought, high-technology surveillance and torture. All that is lacking in its description of the worst-case, long-term scenario of life under a market state is use of the capacity to borrow money and of mass media technology advertising luxury products, to convince people to accept a 'treadmill' consumerist existence. In such a society, 'liberty' may gradually erode into the freedom to purchase, or of a few powerful entrepreneurs to exploit others, instead of a right supporting the capacity of all citizens to view their life's work as a quest for personal and collective meaning.

Students should be given a chance to develop leadership insights from such literary narratives through being required to seek (but not necessarily achieve) publication and dissemination of their own critical analysis of the principles applied in contemporary issues concerning medical professionalism. Spin-off benefits may arise from the manner in which such students eventually go on to more confidently reshape components of domestic and global health care policy, the goals and working practices of health care corporations, record patient stories in clinical histories in the hospital or practice notes, recount them verbally in shift handover, or, less often, in morbidity and mortality meetings, grand rounds or medical journal case notes.

Such methods encourage student clinicians, health care executives and policy-makers to better perceive how they may gradually 'author' coherence in their life narrative between private conscience and the virtues and principles expected to be upheld by a medical or health care professional. By so stimulating the link between individual conscience and the foundational professional and social virtues upon which a professional regulatory system of (specific or 'pinpoint') rules and (general or 'wave-form') principles is built, medical humanities will grow to have a very practical normative role in an 'integrated' professional regulatory system beyond the age of the market state.[4]

This type of approach to professional education involves elements of *hermeneutics* (understanding leading to personal 'engagement'), as well as an emphasis on what can be termed 'reflective equilibrium' in decision-making, involving a striving for integrity associated with personal and professional aspirations, values and principles. It is thus probably best taught in a setting encouraging large-group debates with required minimum attendance levels.

§iii. *The contemplative life and professional leadership*

Many traditions of moral philosophy have highlighted – and continue to emphasise – the regular daily use of psychological techniques such as prayer, contemplation and meditation, often (but not necessarily) in conjunction with a relaxing environment and music, as a means of enhancing mental peace and concentration, as well as cumulatively developing virtue and self-knowledge.

The author, for example, currently commences every lecture before medical or law students with a brief (5 minutes) secular relaxation exercise. This involves (1) a systematic relaxation of muscular tension, (2) an awareness, then slowing of respiration, (3) imagining stress leaving (with each breath out) through points at which the body contacts the chair, (4) witnessing spontaneous thoughts, (5) visualising or imagining a relaxing place, before (6) listening to the outside sounds.

Regular meditative, contemplative and relaxation practices (say in the early morning, or before bed) may also improve work–life balance, assist with coherence decision-making, help with counselling after traumatic resuscitation experiences and aid the treatment of depression and suicidal ideation. In conceptions of medical professionalism beyond the age of the market state, institutional encouragement of such practices is likely to be regarded as just as important as rosters that allow sufficient hours of sleep and rest, regular holidays, and sick days taken without institutional or peer recrimination.

Those in charge of a globally corporatised health care system are unlikely to specifically prohibit (and could even encourage) what may often be viewed as 'quaint' activities focused on contemplation and relaxation, unless they are perceived to 'waste' time, or create attitudes of independent thought and conscience that challenge local management or national policy decisions. Implementation of such strategies, however, may be adversely affected by workplace legislation and contracts allowing employers to limit or prevent activities alleged to interfere with productivity, or by the misunderstanding that such practices represent either a threat to, or a front for, religious ideology.

Viewing familiarity with relaxation and contemplation as a natural part of medical professionalism beyond the age of the market state will complement the 'integrated' regulatory system's foundational emphasis on virtue and conscience. The premise here is that a calm mind is more likely to promote virtue-building applications of principle in the face of obstacles. Integrating such practices into medical professional education will complement that system's requirement for competence in understanding and respecting the diverse range of spiritual and religious belief systems patients bring to the treatment of suffering. It may counteract the instrumental use and proselytising of spiritual and religious philosophies and techniques in clinical decision and health policy-making, which can be deeply offensive to some patients.

Beyond the age of the market state, integrating relaxation and contemplation practices into professional education could even become an important aspect of the scientific exploration of consciousness. Relevant related research questions may include the development of artificial intelligence, the quantum basis of consciousness and its interaction with nanotechnology, understanding brain injury and the possibility of studying consciousness free from any conception of the self.

One intriguing related hypothesis concerns use of the Kantian categorical imperative (that human beings should act according to principles that can be universally applicable) as a subject for daily prayer about personal and professional activities. The proposition thereby tested, by the individual, is that this may facilitate a type of training relationship between his or her conscience (or pure goodwill) and a greater consciousness, capable of altering our perception of matter in time and space to become a progression of opportunities to develop virtue through the consistent application of universally applicable principles in the face of obstacles. Such a view of the way the world works, for those with the capacities to form and learn from such a transcendent relationship, has a plausible resonance with the quantum and relativistic nature of reality revealed by modern science, particulary if not linked with any prescribed religious imagery or ideology. Experimenting with such a philosophy could have profoundly positive implications beyond the era of the market state.

Using this approach, retirement from professional practice would not mean the end of a socially meaningful existence, but the beginning of its culmination, through increased time and inclination to hone contemplative skills. The ultimate benefit of a career lived according to a desire to enhance conscience and virtue will then be experienced as a mind capable of sustained concentration, untroubled by petty vexations and animosities, and increasingly both intrigued and inspired by thoughts of the eternal.

Some might view the stark contrast here as being with the goals and ambitions of the materialist, opportunistically hedonistic or consumerist existence promoted as acceptable for people living in the age of the market state. This would be too simplistic an analysis. The capacity of profit-driven corporate globalisation to sustainably enhance the material conditions of the people of the world is a valuable goal, and many of its leaders would privately embrace spiritual and religious philosophies. A major challenge for innovative educative systems seeking to help medical professional regulation move beyond the era of the market state is to link health care governance, business and policy models not only theoretically with those foundational social and professional virtues that characterise bioethics and international human rights, but also with practical techniques promoting mental calm, harmony and the ability of awareness to consistently act from the vantage point of self-recollection in eternity. If socially powerful leaders of medical professionalism begin by example to show that the essence of human yearning is not consumer desire, that markets need to focus on the ultimate service they are constructed to deliver, their education will have positively facilitated the destiny of nature on Earth in ways that are difficult now to imagine.

Chapter summary and cases for further discussion

- Student health professionals and policy-makers should be taught how the principles of medical professionalism merge with those emerging from the corporate-controlled market state.

- Encouraging such students to develop a commitment in conscience to a wide range of coherent professional principles may be facilitated by a variety of educational techniques.

- Such techniques can include interactive group discussions and encouragement to publish critical analysis, moot health law courts set in ideal 'integrated' regulatory environments, use of humanities literature and training in non-religious meditation and contemplation techniques.

- Use of such contemplative techniques could be linked to a testable post-market state philosophy about living life to develop virtue individually, professionally and socially through the application of universally applicable principles in the face of obstacles.

Case study: Fred's story

A medical student had been talking to an old ex-soldier ('digger') called Fred in a rural hospital. 'He told me he'd been on patrol with an Owen gun in the Stanleys,' said the student, 'when this Jap came round from behind a tree and threw a grenade at him. The grenade blew him to pieces, and he remembered spurting arterial blood. But they got him back to the aid post alive, by using tourniquets. When he woke up, all he could think was, "How wonderful it is not to die when you're young."'[5] What obligations (in terms of life values and ideals to transform into policies) does a generation that has enjoyed a prolonged period of peace have to repay the debt of those who fought and died to achieve it?

Case study: Jason's story

Medical students are exceedingly concerned about a full fee-paying colleague who always seems to be on the spot for sudden, unexplained deaths on the wards. No one really likes him, because although he can seem very friendly, it is soon clear that this is only because he wants to get something. He reacts violently to criticism and is very arrogant in his dismissal of any notions of medical professionalism that aren't focused on profit-earning. One student says, 'We were in this restaurant yesterday when this news item on TV said a security guard had killed 21 people using cyanide. The student said, "There you go – every time I get a good idea, someone beats me to it."'[6] The student's father is a substantial benefactor to the university. What principles should guide how a regulatory system for medical professionalism should handle such a trainee?

4

CORPORATE
INFLUENCE
ON
INSTITUTIONAL
MEDICAL
ETHICS

I. The problems of centralisation and self-regulation

This chapter attempts to critically analyse how 'integrated' medical professionalism, in the era beyond the market state, may reshape increased corporate influence over institutionalised structures supporting medical ethics – professional codes, guidelines, peer review bodies, ethics committees, medical boards, indemnity insurers and health care complaints organisations.

One proposition explored here is that the incorporation of corporate executives and policy-makers into an 'integrated' system of health professional regulation may make it more likely that such ethics stuctures will promote community trust by prioritising collective and individual virtues such as justice, loyalty to the relief of patient suffering and respect for human dignity.

A corollary of this hypothesis is that as 'integrated' professional regulation moves beyond the era of the market state, it will more stringently and effectively restrain ethics centralisation and industry self-regulation – as well as political appointments and corporate user-pays financing. These otherwise may inhibit research and clinical ethics committees, standing bodies for expert ethics guidance and health technology safety and cost-effectiveness regulatory agencies from acting as key forums where the global social contract about health care can be renegotiated, democratised and revitalised.

§i. *Medical professional organisations and leadership*

Self-regulatory clinical governance structures (such as peer review and clinical privileges committees), statutory health complaints organisations, research and clinical ethics committees, medical boards, specialist colleges, professional associations and medical defence insurers often appear to be like the protagonists in Patrick White's novel *Riders in the Chariot*. Although they know about each other's existence, they do not appreciate the significance of their mutual striving to express a common vision (in this case about the ideal form of medical professionalism in a social contract); this lack of communication is detrimental to the sustainability of human society in general.

'Clinical governance' is a term which broadly describes institutional structures designed to improve safety and quality in health care delivery through standard setting, risk management (particularly via peer review and incident monitoring), training, and professional and organisational accountability. As regulation moves beyond a fully privatised health care system, clinical governance may become more a trusted means of protecting public safety than a management and marketing strategy for reducing costs and limiting external criticism of the organisation.

Beyond the age of the market state, medical professional associations operating within an 'integrated' system of professional regulation are more likely to be trusted as the guardians of domestic and global public goods in health care. Yet the history of such associations has shown that they have been extremely effective political lobby groups when it comes to protecting professional incomes, even if that means opposing legislation seeking to improve social justice in health policy. This means, for example, that their spokespeople have often been subject to conflicts of interest when making media pronouncements about privatisation of hospitals and medical education, or pharmaceutical company influence over professional standards. Without thorough institutional reforms reinforcing 'integrated' educational instruction, such associations will continue to have difficulty expressing genuine commitment to the view that a lucrative professional service monopoly is a privilege granted in return for service.

In the post-market state era, specialist medical colleges will continue to establish threshold levels of competence through arduous and exacting postgraduate exams. They will also prepare guidelines concerning contentious areas of clinical practice in their specific area of expertise. Their role will remain critical to maintaining professional standards. However, there may be a need to modify or reverse such specialist colleges' plans to establish or assist courses (with very high fees) for higher degrees in which advanced trainees learn world-class techniques in private facilities, but thereby erode the skills base and ethos of public hospitals. Health corporation executives and policy-makers will be recognised as needing familiarity with specialist training through such colleges.

Medical boards and councils, in the post-market state era, will comprise a mixture of representatives, some elected by a broad range of health professionals and some appointed by government to reflect community interests. Such boards and councils will continue to control admission to medical practice, registration, certification and supervision of standards of practice, with the primary purpose not only of protecting public safety, but also of enhancing and promoting foundational professional virtues such as loyalty to the relief of patient suffering. To this end, they will more transparently and accountably use options including the regulatory 'big stick' of professional misconduct proceedings for conduct reasonably regarded as dishonourable by brethren of good repute and competency, under the overall supervision of a Human Rights Commissioner. Single statutory regimes will increasingly control registration of all health professionals (including health corporation executives and policy-makers). In the post-market state era, such medical boards and councils will become more willing to extend their support for foundational professional virtues into critiques of national and global health policy. Failure to take such roles seriously may see regulatory powers removed from such boards and councils and given instead to independent statutory bodies.

In the present age of the market state, many boardroom drivers of corporate globalisation push for policies of free trade in professional services. This in turn pressures medical boards and specialist medical colleges to loosen restrictions on educational qualifications and standards of competence. One strategy to balance such pressures may be the organisation by medical boards, for public access, of 'report card' information about a physician's or surgeon's level of specialist training and experience, academic qualifications, level of complaints and legal malpractice claims, as well as, most importantly, conflicts of interest from corporate research funding or employment, statistical data on patient load, operative success and failure rates and level of post-operative complications. The argument that many unintended consequences detrimental to health professionals could flow from divulging this sort of knowledge does not adequately take into account either the capacity of improved information technology to facilitate transparency, public safety and trust, or the professional and social virtues that form the foundations of 'integrated' regulation.

The primary task of medical defence insurers in the current age of the market state is to provide medical practitioners with legal representation, advice and indemnity in relation to claims of professional incompetence. This often places such organisations at odds with the role of medical boards to maintain overall ethical standards and protect public safety. This is chiefly because the dominant aims of the insurers have been to increase profit by minimising claim expenditure and to maximise client satisfaction through successful defences. They are one step removed from the system of legal ethics, which emphasises the right of all accused to competent representation.

Medical defence insurers in many nations nonetheless have played an important regulatory role in shaping the content of domestic health law, by deciding which cases to defend and take to appeal. Their presentations and publications are also a major source of legal education for doctors. The large sums of money doctors (and governments in some jurisdictions) pay to such insurers probably promotes both legalism (an overwhelming deference to the regulatory power of law) and free market fundamentalism in health care policy. It promotes, in other words, a system whereby the legal content of professional regulation can be shaped by commercial realities. Only about 40 per cent of indemnity contributions by health professionals actually go to compensating patients who have suffered from adverse incidents during their care. The system so inhibits claimants that only about 1 in 7 of iatrogenically injured patients seeks compensation. Beyond the era of the market state, creation of a global system of no fault compensation for medical error is likely to be much more coherent with 'integrated' professional regulation.

Clinical medical ethicists often make valuable contributions to medical professionalism through their work on regulatory organisations, commissions and committees, and as individual commentators in academic journals, newspapers or other media. The academic independence associated with university employment should place bioethicists (and salaried medical professionals with university appointments) in a secure position from which to critically analyse the impacts of health care privatisation. Many would argue, however, that during the market state era such independence has often faded into a memory, as universities organised as money-making enterprises increasingly lack any genuine commitment to academic independence. Introducing policies that support the role of bioethicists as rigorous commentators on health professional regulation will be an important method, in the post-market state age, of ensuring continued revitalisation of the social contract with the medical knowledge elite.

In a hospital setting, clinical ethics committees will have a stronger role, during the post-market state era, in developing institution-specific guidelines about professional standards. Such a group will increasingly operate as a responsibility diffuser for semi-urgent clinical decisions on matters such as late-term abortions and withdrawal and withholding of treatment. Appointments to these bodies will continue to be voluntary and generally without remuneration, as this promotes objectivity and independence, and sets an influential example of respect for foundational professional virtues. Members will continue to include lawyers and bioethicists, as well as representatives from the profession and the community, but also corporate executives and health policy-makers. This will ensure that the group remains well positioned to reflect on the ideals the community expects the profession, and the health care system in general, to embody.

Some commentators have considered the dominance of physician appointments one reason for an alleged gap between the typical hospital clinical ethics committee and the ideal Rawlsian group of social contractors.[1] But the broad community and professional representation on such committees, as well as their indemnity from legal liability, gives them a strong position from which to 'push back' against local corporate initiatives they perceive as adversely impacting on foundational social and professional virtues. This will be particularly true if they are able to organise and critique health policy at national and international levels.

§ii. Corporate spin and codes of ethics: 'Service of humanity' as a brand name

One of big challenges for medical professionalism in and beyond the era of fully privatised global health care will be whether or not the *Hippocratic Oath* continues to exert any symbolic moral power amongst medical educators, regulators, health corporation executives and health policy-makers. Its call to not just doctors, but health professionals broadly, to 'preserve the purity' of their 'life and art', and its encouragement to practise with 'conscience and dignity', has often come to be regarded, during the era of the market state, as no more than a curious literary flourish; worse, the oath can be seen as a brand name that corporate managers can profitably attach to their health service products.

In the post-market state era, codes of medical ethics are likely to contain more references to medical virtues, conscience and international human rights. Further, they will be less frequently marginalised to accommodate corporate-influenced changes to legal rules. They will most likely include more explicit references to their role of assisting health professionals to morally calibrate, for example, statutory definitions of professional misconduct in registration or licensing legislation. Their explicit references to health care 'consumers' will be gradually replaced by the term 'patients', chiefly on the ground that the latter term affords the vulnerable ill a greater range of protections and is more likely to evoke beneficial traditional professional virtues.

Emphasis on loyalty to the relief of patient suffering in such codes will no longer be denigrated by the relevant business managers as causing harmful conflicts with cost-cutting and profit-maximising measures, or being out of step with the contemporary physician's role as gatekeeper for the market forces and economic realities of managed care plans. Corporate health managers will be less likely to announce, for example, that such professional regulatory bodies must now have a more realistic view of what level of altruism can be achieved by doctors subscribing to diverse moral philosophies while employed by organisations seeking to maximise shareholder returns. Professional virtues in codes of medical ethics will be less frequently presented by such corporate managers as an unnecessary intrusion on the personal morality and choice of consumers.

Finally, in the post-market state era, the taking of a public oath or the making of a 'profession' – upon graduation, or admission to practice – of commitment to traditional professional virtues and ethical principles will become a more important aspect of the professional regulatory system. Making such a statement will be promoted as crucial to the process of incorporating those values into the life narrative of the doctors concerned. It will be more widely regarded as the culmination of education in medical professionalism and leadership. Many students may start with a template such as the *Geneva Declaration*, and then make whatever alterations they agree constitute the duties central to their professional conscience. In a society seeking sustainability, the acquisition of virtue will become a paramount consideration.

§iii. *Conscientious disobedience and whistleblowing: Governance threats to the market state*

In his short story *A Case History*, Chekhov writes of a house physician sent by his professor to visit the ill daughter of a mill owner in a provincial town. The family thinks the young girl is near death from some insidious physical complaint. The young doctor, however, diagnoses severe anxiety and depression. Accepting an invitation to stay the night before returning, he inspects the huge factory and sees the hopeless faces of the workers. Overwhelmed by the brutality of their slavery, he recognises that, similarly, conscience must have been awakened in this sensitive young lady. He comforts her, explaining that feelings of loneliness and despair are natural for one in this situation.

As discussed earlier, the Nazi doctors' trial after World War II led to the core duties of medical professionalism being reaffirmed through codes such as the *Nuremberg Declaration*, the *Geneva Declaration* and the *International Code of Medical Ethics*. All of these supported the ethical duty of physicians to make conscience-based decisions for the patient's good, if need be, in disobedience of legal rules. Codes of medical ethics have supported this radical strain of what may be termed normative calibration, advocating potential conscientious disobedience to laws, as being at the heart of professional regulation. The American Medical Association, for example, in its introduction to opinions on its *Code of Medical Ethics*, states:

> [E]thical obligations typically exceed legal duties. In some cases the law mandates unethical conduct. In general, when physicians believe a law is unjust, they should work to change the law. In exceptional circumstances of unjust laws, ethical responsibilities should supersede legal obligations.[2]

The British Medical Association, similarly, declares that doctors should not necessarily consider that legalisation of conduct makes it permissible professionally from an ethical point of view:

> If the law were to change to permit doctors to end patients' lives on request, participation in assisted suicide would be a matter for the individual doctor's conscience, subject to professional guidance issued by the regulatory body.[3]

The Australian Medical Association, in its Ethical Code, also supports the need for medical professionals to maintain the capacity for independent analysis of their legal obligations against moral and ethical norms related to the care of patients:

> In order to provide high quality healthcare, you must safeguard
> clinical independence and professional integrity from increased
> demands from society, third parties, individual patients and
> governments ... Recognise your right to refuse to carry out
> services which you consider to be professionally unethical,
> against your moral convictions, imposed on you for either
> administrative reasons or for financial gain or which you
> consider are not in the best interest of the patient.[4]

The Canadian Medical Association, in its Code of Medical Ethics,
highlights the need for health professionals to be competent in the type
of coherence reasoning advocated here for 'integrated' professional
regulation:

> Physicians may experience tension between different
> ethical principles, between ethical and legal or regulatory
> requirements, or between their own ethical convictions and
> the demands of other parties. Training in ethical analysis and
> decision-making during undergraduate, postgraduate and
> continuing medical education is recommended for physicians
> to develop their knowledge, skills and attitudes needed to deal
> with these conflicts. Consultation with colleagues, regulatory
> authorities, ethicists, ethics committees or others who have
> relevant expertise is also recommended.[5]

Laws permitting or even requiring medical complicity in torture or
capital punishment represent acute examples of such tensions with
basic ethical norms and with those of international human rights.
One high-profile case occurred in South Africa under apartheid rule.
In 1977 the political activist Steve Biko was detained without warrant
or prospect of trial under South African anti-terrorism legislation.
He was beaten by security police and suffered a massive intracerebral
haemorrhage.[6] None of the doctors who saw Biko offered treatment,
or would subsequently admit that he had been tortured. One doctor
at the inquiry into Biko's death said he thought Biko was 'shamming'.
Here is an excerpt of Biko's barrister's questioning of that doctor:

> Did you think that extensor plantar reflex could be shammed?
>
> *No.*

Do you think a man could sham red blood cells in the cerebral spinal fluid?

No.

In terms of the *Hippocratic Oath*, to which, I take it, you subscribe, are not the interests of your patients paramount?

Yes.

But in this instance they were subordinated to the interests of security. Is that a fair statement?

Yes. I didn't know in this particular situation one could override decisions made by responsible police officers.

Where global health care is controlled by market states, a variety of laws that tend to favour corporate profits can be passed; they do not necessarily favour the interests of patients or public health in general. Some of these laws restrict an important role of health professionals in the area of basic principles of institutional medical ethics: informing and warning the public directly of health care risks, despite contrary contractual obligations (whistleblowing).

In 1999 Dr Koos Stiekema, for example, an employee with the multinational pharmaceutical company Organon, disputed the safety of its clinical trial of pentasaccharide as an anticoagulant in unstable angina. Stiekema claimed that his research had established that doses lower than 4mg would be ineffective, but the company planned to include a dose of 2.5mg from the outset. After arbitration failed, Stiekema took his concerns to the independent ethics committees overseeing the study. When the trial was finally published, without any apparent excess deaths, the company sued Stiekema for causing delay and lost profits by breaching his contractual confidentiality agreement with it. At first instance damages were awarded, but this was overturned on appeal, the Amsterdam court finding that his breaching the confidentiality clause was 'justified by a higher interest'.[7]

Whistleblowing has emerged as one of the most successful quality and safety interventions in contemporary health care. Far from being ostracised by their professional colleagues, in the post-market state era, health care whistleblowers will *prima facie* be supported as professionals attempting to demonstrate commitment to foundational professional virtues principles in difficult circumstances.[8] Corporate attempts to undermine the regulatory role of health care whistleblowing by contractual restrictions on staff contacting media will be overcome in a general and even pre-emptive sense by legislation that more effectively protects public interest disclosures and by policies that facilitate joint academic appointments.

Whistleblowers will be more effectively protected from reprisal (especially if such reprisals are disguised as performance reviews) when they have followed established channels in making a public interest disclosure after attempting unsuccessfully to protect patient and public safety via internal clinical governance pathways. This will send an influential signal to the general community that a health care institution or organisation working within a professional regulatory system expects its staff to prioritise conscience and loyalty to the relief of patient suffering.

II. Guidelines and clinical pathways as corporate directives

§i. Corporate self-governance and responsibility: Outsourcing professionalism

Beyond the era of the market state, specific guidance on contentious areas of medical ethics and professional responsibilities will continue to be provided through guidelines produced by statutory authorities, commissions or standing committees with ministerially appointed experts. Key issues will include research on human subjects, assisted reproductive technology, brain death, organ donation both during life and afterwards, genetic testing and the use of new technologies in health care and medical research.

Such professional guidelines are not law at the moment, but they are often used in professional adjudication to determine right or wrong conduct and, upon breach, permit self-regulatory sanctions such as loss of employment or competitive grant funding, and/or admission to remedial programs. Further, insofar as guidelines help define professional standards of care, their breach may eventually precipitate, or assist in the determination of, legal proceedings. The regulatory importance of guidelines makes it critical for medical professionalism that appointments to the bodies enunciating them are carefully scrutinised for conflicts of interest.

Professional guidelines should be distinguished from practice protocols, allocation guidelines, clinical pathways, or clinical algorithms, all of which are self-regulation instruments prepared by corporate and public health care managers.

Doctors and patients have often been told that the main role of such instruments is to improve service through raising and creating greater institutional uniformity in the standard of care, improving technical proficiency and the practical conduct of research projects. Their proponents claim they reduce costly individuality in the provision of medical care (particularly in the requesting of expensive diagnostic tests) and limit institutional legal liability. They are also promoted as enhancing consumer trust by identifying, clarifying and requiring communication of physician options before procedures are agreed to and undertaken. Compliance with them is ensured by threat of employment termination, demotion or lack of advancement.

Such pathways and algorithms have also become a means of imposing corporate values on the practice of medicine. They can be viewed as providing financial disincentives or incentives for physicians to acquiesce in a subthreshold standard of care for profit-maximising reasons. They also risk abusing patient trust by limiting the diagnostic testing or therapeutic options of doctors while gagging the latter's capacity to reveal such restrictions to patients. Institutes of company directors often argue that without generating trust among investors, companies and their shareholders, sustainability of profits is not achievable. The Dow Jones Sustainability World Index shows that health care companies represent six of the top twenty. The Global Reporting Initiative (GRI) Sustainability Reporting Guidelines, produced in collaboration with the United Nations' Environment Program, have been promoted as a means by which potential investors can correlate a company's sustainability with its ethical performance. Such initiatives show that corporate responsibility in the health care sector could be conceived as involving commitment to foundational virtues, much in the way that such beneficial traits can be ascribed to collective entities such as professions or societies. In the post-market state era, the legitimacy of corporate health care practice guidelines is likely to suffer if their development continues to be characterised by insufficient prior public and professional consultation and their content by inadequate reference to related professional norms in institutional medical ethics and international human rights.

§ii. Corporate influence over research ethics

The vices of sloth, vainglory and avarice are likely to remain considerable threats to patient safety and respect for dignity as long as humanity is constituted as it is. Historical examples of unethical conduct in scientific research will continue to echo in dilemmas and scandals in the post-market state era. Of lasting relevance will be Henry Beecher's landmark review of lack of informed consent, which revealed, amongst other things, a clinical trial where antibiotics known to be effective were withheld from the placebo arm to improve the credibility of data.[9] Also providing continuing lessons will be the Tuskegee Syphilis Study (in which physicians ensured that 400 African-Americans remained an untreated control group), the Willowbrook hepatitis study, and the New Zealand clinical trial in which women with cervical cancer underwent observation rather than therapy.

In the era of the market state, public disclosure of scientific truth creates profound tensions with the interests of corporate health care managers, causing fluctuations in share price, flights of investment capital and an undermining of consumer confidence. In 2006, for example, the ironically named ILLUMINATE clinical trial of a compound combining two anti-cholesterol drugs (torcetrapib and atorvastatin [the latter's patent was soon to expire]) was discontinued because of an apparent excess of subject mortality and cardiovascular events in the trial's treatment arm. This reduced the stock value of the Pfizer pharmaceutical company by 11 per cent (over A$30 billion) and led to speculation that it would launch a takeover bid for another multinational pharmaceutical organisation with better 'pipeline' prospects for new products.

Perhaps the greatest contemporary quest by the medical profession for scientific truth was the Human Genome Project (HGP). It is hardly surprising that it became a race between health professionals espousing differing philosophies concerning private rights, public goods and the role of research ethics.

When the HGP was established, 3 per cent of its initial $200 million of public funding was allocated to study related ethical, legal and social issues (ELSI) and prepare guidelines on them. Many of the resultant academic publications attempted to create new regulatory principles for this explosion of human genetic knowledge. That output often appeared to have little to recommend it but more memory-friendly alliteration: counselling, consent, choice, control, confidentiality and competence, or even communication, collaboration, compensation, continual review and (no) conflict of interest. Devised in the absence of justifying empirical data and rapidly, without prolonged analysis or the attempt to achieve coherence with an interpretive tradition of professional principle or international human rights, such 'created' ethical principles appear to have generally contributed little more than the satisfaction of grant requirements.

On the other hand, guidelines that used many sources – including the UNESCO *Universal Declaration on the Human Genome and Human Rights*, the World Health Organization (WHO), the Human Genome Organisation (HUGO), the International Council of Science Unions, national ethics committees and commissions – successfully contributed to a prohibition on research into germ line gene therapy, human reproductive cloning and the creation of animal–human hybrid beings. Attempts to use such guidelines as a regulatory strategy to make the human genome the common heritage of humanity and to protect it from corporate exploitation (particularly through patents over research) are likely to more successful in the post-market state era.

In the age of the market state, researchers under pressure from grant commercialisation requirements, or involvement on the boards of biotech companies, to push ahead with such a potentially lucrative area need to rapidly establish the clinical efficacy of new health technologies. To do so and to advance their careers, they experience increasing temptation, in a dominantly privatised health care system, to overstate their success. Scientific fraud might be only one outcome of such pressure.[10]

A dominant model in the market state era is that once new health technologies are developed, clinical trials have to be organised with an eye to marketing strategy, as well as safety and efficacy evaluation. Inducements, financial or otherwise (access to therapy that would otherwise be too expensive, for instance), may be offered, in such circumstances, by private clinical trial organising companies to the poor or needy to participate in inherently risky research studies.[11] Although principles of research ethics require disclosure of conflicts of interest in such circumstances, very often this does not occur.[12]

In the 1960s, the Australian obstetrician William McBride and the German Widukind Lenz began associating phocomelia or 'seal limbs' in babies with maternal consumption of thalidomide. Because FDA safety regulator Frances Kelsey, strictly following institutional guidelines of scientific ethics emphasising the 'precautionary principle', was dissatisfied with data presented by Richardson-Merrell Inc., the drug was never marketed in the United States. McBride achieved fame for his discovery, but his later work attempting to show birth defects caused by imipramine and debenox was found to have involved scientific fraud.

It would be a tragedy, once scientific research begins to make frontier technologies such as gene therapy and nanotherapeutics a reality, if the lessons from such case studies have to be repeated. This is less likely to occur if medical research ethics is drawn systematically into the type of 'integrated' and sustainable professional regulatory system advocated here.

Beyond the age of the market state, institutional forms of medical ethics will more uniformly reinforce the understanding that many governance issues will be resolved if professionals are encouraged to make accurate decisions by moving past the habitual inadequacies of their own thinking. These include fears, prejudices, misconceptions and the inability to trust in the the tangible benefits of shaping their professional life and art towards virtue.

Chapter summary and cases for further discussion

- The ethics of medical professionalism are institutionalised through a variety of codes, guidelines, protocols and clinical pathways, administered by clinical governance structures, medical registration boards, professional associations, specialist colleges, expert committees and indemnity insurers.

- All these institutional forms of medical ethics are susceptible to corporate influence in the age of the market state, and are not uniformly focused on loyalty to relief of patient suffering.

- One marker of the level of commitment institutional medical ethics has to foundational social and professional virtues will be the respect and protection it accords those who make public interest disclosures.

- In the age of the market state, the discretionary ethics of corporate responsibility cannot be relied upon to consistently protect the interests of patients or health professionals, particularly in areas such as scientific research.

- In the post-market state era, institutional medical ethics will have a much more explicit role in assisting health professionals to calibrate norms of law relevant to patient care.

Case study: Jason's story

A medical student saw a young patient called Jason, swollen and yellow with multi-system disease from binge drinking. Jason had joined Alcoholics Anonymous and was on the transplant list. He had a grossly distended abdomen, but the student's team decided not to give Jason an ascites tap due to the very low clotting capacity of his blood (caused by liver disease). The student later said, 'I last saw him on Friday afternoon. He'd taken a slight downturn and was being managed conservatively. When I turned up for the Monday morning round, Jason's room was being cleaned out and the bed had been changed. The nursing staff said he'd died over the weekend. His care had been transferred to another team. On advice from the new treating physician, the weekend registrar, in disregard of our written warnings in the patient notes, performed an abdominal tap. Despite blood transfusions and pressure bandaging, over the course of the weekend, the patient had slowly bled to death. We interns were told not to attend the quality assurance (QA) meeting. I asked why not and was told that certain physicians didn't want us knowing about "things that go wrong". Some senior clinicians feared we would blab about their "bad" cases and disregard their professional abilities if we were aware of them. We'd be allowed to attend QAs after a few months, when we "got the hang of things".'[13] How should an 'integrated' professional regulatory system best respond to the issues in this story?

Case study: Jeremy's story

Jeremy, an intern, was working in the Emergency Department (ED) of a private rural hospital when a patient was admitted suffering a stab wound to the heart. The patient had lost all vital signs moments before he arrived in the trauma bay. A check of online medical records showed the patient was underinsured for 'catastrophic' cover. The ED registrar, who was very busy, said, 'This consumer is dead; leave him dead.' Jeremy disobeyed the hospital's practice protocols, got the rib spreaders, opened the chest, removed a large clot from the pericardium and sutured the laceration to the myocardium. The patient's vital signs returned and after a dose of thiopentone (to decrease cerebral requirements for oxygen) he was taken to the operating theatre. The patient survived to walk out of the hospital. Jeremy was criticised in the grand rounds presentation of the case, but not by all.[14] How should a clinical ethics committee, or medical board, evaluate the potential tension between institutional principles of ethics and legal obligations in this case?

5

HEALTH
LAW
AS A
CORPORATE
MARKETING
STRATEGY

I. Medical malpractice and system error

§i. Beyond health law at the service of corporate interests

In the era of the market state, judicial rulings and legislation creating health law have been increasingly influenced by ideologically based judicial appointments, the capacity of industry to fund protracted litigation, as well as prior intense lobbying of Ministers. The tendency has been to make health law resemble a marketing or profit-making strategy implemented by the managers of multinational corporations and their allies in government.

In *Garcetti v Ceballos* (547 US (2006)), for example, a narrow majority in the US Supreme Court held that government employees' job-related disclosures were not protected by constitutional human rights guarantees of freedom of speech, regardless of the extent to which they were attempting to protect public health and safety. It was predicted that the ruling would have a chilling effect on the willingness of public employees to risk their livelihoods to expose, for example, fraud and waste in government contracts with the private sector, and would hinder efforts of whistleblowers to reveal related incompetence or maladministration.[1]

Similarly, in the *Chaoulli* case ([2005] 1 SCR 791, 2005 SCC 35) a narrow majority of judges on the Supreme Court of Canada found that a prohibition on private health insurance in Quebec legislation violated the rights of patients under section 1 of the Quebec *Charter of Human Rights and Freedoms*. This declares that 'Every human being has a right to life, and to personal security, inviolability and freedom.' A similar argument under the closely related section 7 of the Canadian *Charter of Rights and Freedoms* was rejected. The four majority justices ruled that while the ban on private health insurance in Quebec was designed to protect the integrity of the public health system, it did not mean that patients must endure delays that increased risks of mortality and morbidity. They rejected evidence that private health insurance would lead to an eventual demise of public health care in Quebec. The decision was widely viewed as somewhat naïve in its understanding of the objectives and strategies of corporate globalisation and reckless in encouraging (without a democratic mandate) health care privatisation in Canada.

In 2006, in the Chennai High Court, the pharmaceutical manufacturer Novartis challenged the refusal by a patent office in India to accord intellectual property protection to its new brand-name medication Gleevec. The patent office had ruled that the drug (for the treatment of myeloid leukaemia) was not sufficiently 'innovative': under section 3(d) of the Indian *Patents Act*, it did not result from the enhancement of the known efficacy of a substance, or the discovery of any new property or new use. Novartis argued, through its lawyers, that the Indian Parliament was not allowed by the WTO TRIPs agreement to pass legislation linking patentability of new pharmaceuticals with a definition of 'inventive step' that excluded minor molecular modifications of limited clinical efficacy. Novartis pleaded that the legislation should be amended; otherwise, they said, once the appeals and dispute resolution processes were exhausted, trade sanctions would be enforced. Their opponents argued, amongst other things, that the right to life in section 21 of the Indian Constitution included a right to health which would be breached if the drug company succeeded in its strategy to limit generic competition. The annual price of generic treatment per patient for Gleevec used to be US$2100; the Novartis price is US$26,000.

The *Medicare Prescription Drug Improvement and Modernization Act* 2003 (US) is another instructive example. It was originally promoted as a measure that would help senior citizens and people with disabilities cope with rising US health care costs, through measures such as allowing the importing of cheaper medicines from Canada. Instead, lobbying by an army of corporate officials (numbering almost double the number of congressmen and senators they regularly met with) ensured that its provisions created a vast subsidy for brand-name medicines. The resultant so-called Medicare Part D gave elderly patients a choice of hundreds of insurance plans and created a 'donut' hole of no government coverage for citizens on low incomes. It prevented the US Federal government from 'interfering' by using its bulk buying power for Medicare beneficiaries to negotiate medicines prices on cost-effectiveness criteria (as the Australian and South Korean governments do and US states can do by pooling their preferred drug lists). The statute also authorised a study to ascertain the alleged financial damage sustained by US corporations and citizens as a result of pharmaceutical price controls in OECD (Organization for Economic Co-operation and Development) countries.

This chapter considers how the content and process of global health law can tame such corporate influence within an 'integrated' system of medical professional regulation. To do this, it attempts to imagine how the content of different areas of health law will operate beyond the age of the market state. The age of the market state, as previously mentioned, represents a condition of synergistic relationships between government and private industry in which the latter's goal of achieving profit has a tendency (if not restrained by regulation) to practically supplant efforts to achieve broader social and professional virtues. It is a global ideology supplanting traditional conceptions of capitalism and communism, and like the concept of a social contract, it provides a valuable reference point for arguments about the future of global health policy and practice.

In what we may term the era of the market state, statutory and/or judge-made (common) law has created a tortuous mechanism whereby a few patients injured as a result of medical malpractice could seek compensation. The system has been a profitable one for private law firms and indemnity insurers, but is generally very slow, somewhat unpredictable and involves considerable up-front expenditure by claimants with the risk (if the claim fails) of paying the other side's costs as well as various disbursements and court fees, even in a 'no win–no fee' situation. The bulk of patients so injured never use this system and so receive no compensation.

In the post-market state era, this legalistic approach to compensation for injury arising from medical error is likely to be generally accepted as too slow and capricious (or 'lottery-like'), but also expensive and ill directed in terms of ensuring patient safety. It is unlikely to be acceptable, under the medical profession's renegotiated place in the global social contract, for about 50 per cent of doctors' medical malpractice premiums to compensate only the most severely injured patients, the rest being spent on insurance administration costs and legal fees. In increasing numbers of jurisdictions, 'no fault' legislative compensation schemes will be developed as an alternative remedy, one that is presumptively more coherent with empiric social science research.

Beyond the era of the market state, health laws will be less likely to emerge as lobbied-for strategies to promote corporate profits – this aim may perhaps be slightly ameliorated or obfuscated (chiefly for public relations purposes) by social responsibility and philanthropic initiatives coming from, and well advertised by, those same corporations. Such comments should not be viewed as a gratuitous denigration of all corporations presently involved in health care. They are merely one realistic appraisal of the long-term consequences of the core fiduciary obligations of directors to shareholders, on the one hand, and increasing awareness by greater numbers of citizens of the limited democratic legitimacy behind market fundamentalism in health policy, on the other. The proposal here aims to enhance both the sustainability and the responsibility of such corporations by including them and their senior management within an 'integrated' system of professional regulation that strives to actualise foundational social and professional virtues.

§ii. *The medical duty to rescue*

With the process of coherence reasoning in mind, let us examine how global health law may interact with a medical duty to rescue in a post-market state age. Rescue is perhaps the most virtue-laden context in which a doctor–patient relationship may be commenced. The medical duty to rescue was traditionally considered to be attached to moral and ethical rules. As the era of the market state has progressed, the duty has increasingly become associated with judge-made legal rules and statutory obligations. The decision of the NSW Supreme Court in *Lowns v Woods*[2] was one of the first in a common law jurisdiction to make the medical duty to rescue a legal obligation.[3]

It is a strong social contract argument that a moral principle encouraging rescue should be part of any professional regulatory system which the community expects to be fundamentally characterised by virtues such as competence, caring and compassion, as encompassed within loyalty to the relief of patient suffering. Yet the act of rescuing a stranger necessarily involves justifiable selectivity – the rescuee's resources, training and the danger to himself or herself, as well as others. Hence, it could be argued, a moral or institutional ethical principle requiring rescue by health professionals and policy-makers is unsuitable for conversion into a legal rule, at least without the benefits of extensive debate and clearly legislated exceptions.

In a broader sense, a duty to rescue (for health professionals, including health care corporate executives and policy-makers) will increasingly be conceptualised as part of a state's duty to come to the aid of vulnerable populations, for example by legislation respecting, protecting and fulfilling the preconditions for health or access to health services.[4] A constitutional right to emergency medical treatment (such as that in section 27(3) of the *South African Constitution 1996*) likewise will be viewed as an acceptable policy limit to health care privatisation and an important means of maintaining citizen engagement with the prominent institutions of society.[5]

Legal rules supporting a general medical duty to rescue individuals might appear to similarly support foundational professional and social virtues, while providing a valuable regulatory balance against contrary profit-seeking influences in health care systems. Yet if such legal obligations to rescue are not carefully drafted, they may actually promote intricate avoidance behaviour by busy doctors, or health care managers, fearful of liability. Such provisions, for example, would need to include protections from liability for medical practitioners reasonably involved in 'good Samaritan acts'. A legal obligation on health professionals to rescue individuals could also endanger public safety, if it is not made coherent with specialist college guidelines based on scientific research showing that patient safety is better ensured by immediate retrieval to an appropriate hospital.

Corporate health care managers may suggest that legal rules supporting a medical duty to rescue individuals should be restricted to imposing enforceable obligations upon those professionals and health care organisations whose primary public-advertised role is to undertake such a task: a statutory public rescue body, an Emergency Department, or an ambulance or aeromedical retrieval service, for example. This argument, however, will have to answer criticism that it will be difficult for these organisations to maintain their high-profile association with foundational professional and social virtues, even if subjected to such a legal obligation, if they become privatised and profitability becomes their dominant practical concern.

§iii. *Medical negligence and systems error*

A child in the Emergency Department said, 'I've broken my funny bone.' The intern, who prided himself on meticulous examination skills, couldn't feel a radial pulse. The registrar, however, said he could, and told the intern to do a closed reduction and put on a plaster cast. But the intern couldn't stop thinking a mistake was being made. He ignored the hospital protocols, rang theatre and demanded the patient be taken for an open reduction. The surgeon found the artery had been kinked over a fragment from the supracondylar fracture of the child's left humerus. The registrar was furious when he found out.

The intern probably learnt two things from this incident. First, that clinical excellence and a strong conscience make a valuable combination. Second, that the hidden culture of institutional medicine requires that leaders never be seen to make mistakes. Such an ethos of perfectionism causes many who aspire to leadership roles in the profession, at either clinical, management or policy levels, to deny that their workplace conduct ever produces errors, or to deflect responsibility for proven occurrences. This can create great pressure on junior medical staff, for whom error is a natural part of the learning experience and who often find themselves blamed for adverse incidents that in fact were due more to lack of supervision and institutional support than to lack of knowledge or of commitment to quality and safety in service delivery.

In the era of the market state, malpractice cases are the standard, albeit seriously flawed, mechanism for allowing patients to recover compensation for damage caused to them by medical mistreatment or misdiagnosis. The system has continued long after its flaws have been exposed, in large part because it is perceived by knowledge elites with a strong influence over health policy (private plaintiff lawyers and medical indemnity insurers) to be valuable to their profit-making.

The first conceptual step towards achieving a remedy through this mechanism is to obtain a legal opinion about whether or not the issues fall within a judicially accepted duty of care. If they do, the next is to acquire evidence both proving failure to meet the requisite professional standard of care or skill and resultant damage.

Inevitably these are 'hard' cases for all regulatory participants. This does not mean that there is no settled legal rule to dictate the judicial decision, either because of rule ambiguity, or because the issue is one of first impression. Rather, adjudicative difficulty frequently arises (in those cases not settled out of court) because of implicit, strongly conflicting social and professional principles. Further, judges in medical negligence cases are increasingly perceived as needing to mould their decision beyond the legally represented parties, to a wider regulatory framework designed to prevent recurrence and protect patient safety. This is a challenge that not all judges desire, or are able with equal facility to rise to.

The legal standard of care in cases concerning medical diagnosis and treatment is usually determined by a court using what is termed the standard of the reasonably competent member of the profession. Courts consider expert evidence about current medical knowledge, actual circumstances and any 'holding out' by the defendant of specialist training, or special risks.

The general legal principle is that all patients are owed the same minimum standard of care or skill, regardless of available institutional resources or level of professional qualifications or experience. Where a doctor cannot meet that standard, he or she is required to either not go to work, request advice or assistance, or refer the patient to a colleague. Such a rule places considerable pressure on public-funded, increasingly under-resourced 'safety net' or 'second tier' hospitals.

In the era of the market state, more and more legislation limits corporate liability, and minimises insurance payouts not only for the negligence of employee doctors, but also for defects in the health care products. Caps have been placed on the amount of damages. Periods in which legal claims have to be made have been reduced. Incentives to out of court settlement have been created and the standard of care has been restricted to one that could be satisfied by proof of conformity with practice of even a minority of reasonably competent practitioners. One unsubstantiated policy argument used to justify such legislation has been that the high costs of privatised health care are due to excessive and unnecessary litigation.

In the future, increased human genome information may put significant pressure upon judges and legislators to develop new tortious medical duties of care related to diagnosis and treatment. These are likely to create many costly liability issues and consequent reorganisations of service delivery, as society attempts to fashion sustainability out of its prior addiction to profit above all else.

Particular instances of such problems could involve increased levels of parent-initiated wrongful birth and wrongful pregnancy claims, as well as wrongful life actions brought on behalf of a child negligently damaged *in utero*. A baby born with a genetic defect which could have been discovered by a corporation's patented pre-natal genetic tests, for example, may have a tortious claim against both the test manufacturer and the doctors involved. Recently, the High Court of Australia, for example, decided that damages were recoverable by parents for the cost of raising a healthy child born because of medical negligence in attempting a tubal ligation.[6] The court then decided, in a different case, that damages were not recoverable by a child born with severe disabilities as a result of a doctor's failure to diagnose maternal rubella during pregnancy.[7]

In the post-market state age, decision-makers using an 'integrated' approach to professional regulation are likely to attempt to set instances of alleged medical negligence in their structural or institutional context, rather than focusing on individual blame. This is a logical outcome of coherence reasoning that will encourage health policy-makers, for example, to replace tort law's largely inefficient negative deterrence function with positive institutional change that restricts adverse impacts on public safety. This could include recommendations to implement enterprise enterprise liability, non fault-based patient compensation and non litigation-based dispute resolution mechanisms.

A related judicial approach may involve the extension of direct tortious liability for medical negligence to the corporate owner of a private-funded hospital. This would be premised on the latter's responsibilities to create a safe system of care.[8] Such a tortious duty is likely to require that a corporate hospital manager not only adequately employ, equip and train doctors, but appropriately supervise and provide them with requisite resources and conditions of work.

§iv. Patient abandonment in the market state

In the dark comedy novel *The House of God* (by Samuel Shem, MD), a hospital's overworked junior medical staff seek to limit the number and duration of their professional responsibilities. They do so by 'turfing' or abandoning patients without valid clinical reason to other sub-specialties, after appropriately 'buffing' the charts to protect themselves from litigation.

As a matter of generally applicable ethical and legal rules, the doctor–patient relationship may be ended by mutual consent, expressly by the patient, or by the doctor; but only after reasonable notice and after continuity of care has been ensured by that physician.

Legal rules prohibiting the abandoning of a patient are likely to have created many 'hard' cases within the conceptual model posited here as a fully privatised global health care system. This may be particularly so in relation to the treatment of patients with chronic and untreatable illness, or forms of suffering for which rapid pharmacological treatment is not readily available (for example, many genetic diseases and conditions such as chronic fatigue syndrome). In the age of the market state, pressures naturally arise for factors such as a patient's poverty, or lack of insurance, to be used by corporate managers as a ground for transfer (probably under a more benign description) to other hospitals, as well as delay in, or withdrawal of, care. Such patient 'dumping' or abandonment represents a clear conflict with the principles of an 'integrated' professional regulatory system, and requires a strong response from leading physicians and health policy-makers. This is not always forthcoming.

Beyond the age of the market state, legal rules prohibiting medical abandonment are likely to be reconceptualised by health lawyers and policy-makers as supporting, in practical ways, the fundamental principle that vulnerable patients should not have their trust spurned or exploited. If such a case is proven, the creation of legal rules that facilitate the potential award of substantial damages against corporate managers for creating an unsafe system of care (so-called enterprise medical liability[9]) is one means whereby a legislature and/or judiciary can emphasise its support of fundamental professional virtues and principles.

International human rights will become more relevant to shaping the legal responsibilities of medical professionals in related contexts: prisoners being denied prompt medical assistance can be seen as in violation of Article 7 of the *ICCPR*,[10] and abandonment because of HIV/AIDS infection may be interpreted as a breach of the right to be protected from discrimination.[11]

II. Consent: Trust and the human right to inviolability

§i. *Equality of consent: Convenient fiction?*

In the age of the market state, the reluctance of doctors to take patient consent seriously may be taken to have challenged the legitimacy of that profession's claims to continue as a socially privileged knowledge elite. Politicians dedicated to promoting corporate interests from within the power structures of the market state have gained an apparent public relations legitimacy from the badge of election, their policies being represented as the will of the people. A similar legitimacy has been accorded many health professionals and privatised health care institutions, from the convenient fiction of consumer consent to medical treatment.

In Mikail Bulgakov's story *The Steel Windpipe*, a young doctor endures a blizzard to attend a patient in a remote community. He finds a young girl resembling a 'chocolate box angel' with a pale lilac complexion. She is asphyxiating from the tonsilar membranes of diphtheria. He wishes to perform a tracheostomy, but the grandmother fiercely refuses to allow him to 'cut the girl's throat'. He ignores this objection and proceeds with the emergency procedure. The anatomy is distorted. He despairs of locating the 'windpipe', remembers the mother, makes a final attempt and finds it. The tracheal rings are almost torn out by a fainting assistant, but final success is attained. The operation makes his reputation. In similar vein is the story *Use of Force* by William Carlos Williams, in which a doctor overcomes a young girl's vehement refusal to obtain a view of dangerous diphtheria on her tonsils. 'The damn little brat must be protected against her own idiocy,' cries the exasperated doctor as he inserts the spatula.

The valiant and heroic paternalism implicit in these examples risked becoming something of a historical anachronism in the age of corporate sovereignty over global public health. The dual threats of loss of employment through breach of practice guidelines and malpractice litigation have tended to have a chilling effect on such courageous, conscience-laden 'rescue' (and 'loyalty-affirming') clinical decision-making.

It is likely to remain a general legal rule in most nations that where medical treatment involving physical contact has taken place without patient consent, the situation is similar to that of any other assault. Criminal proceedings result from apprehended conduct allegedly causing fear about the use of, or the actual use of, unlawful physical force, as well as from false imprisonment. Subsequent failure of treatment, however, has been held not to convert what was otherwise a consensual treatment into an assault.

These legal rules are quite ancient. As early as 1329, for example, the English common law held that a legal action for trespass to the person could not be sustained where an oculist, undertaking to heal an eye with herbs, had failed.[12] Similar cases were *Stratton v Swanlond* (1374: a surgeon who undertook to heal a traumatised hand only made it septic[13]) and *Skyrne v Butolf* (1388: a leech was paid and contracted to cure a man of ringworms, but failed[14]).

Since to be actionable, the degree of such unlawful force need only be minimal, a patient's claim of mere touching by a medical practitioner without consent has often sufficed. Medical motive is irrelevant, provided the act itself appears intentional or reckless. The absence of hostility towards the patient provides no defence. A doctor's mistaken belief that there was consent (even if such a belief were unreasonable) offers protection from a charge of criminal assault, but would not necessarily defeat civil liability under tort law.

Courts have been prepared to infer, imply or reject consent from the conduct of the patient and surrounding circumstances (such as waiting in an emergency department cubicle, or extending an arm for an injection). Allegations of assault or battery are difficult to substantiate as the patient bears the onus of proving that the apprehension or application of force occurred without consent. Necessity and the need to prevent imminent risk of severe injury may justify a doctor's proceeding wihout patient consent, provided this is coherent with relevant ethics and human rights principles.

A classic lack of consent dilemma involves a surgeon making a decision to remove or alter tissue – issues not previously discussed with the patient – during an operation. In the German *Myom* case, for example, a hysterectomy was performed without prior consent in an operation to remove a muscular tumour.[15] In the Swedish decision of *Kerstin*, a patient was told surgeons were to 'loosen up' the tissue around a nerve producing hip pain. Instead they deliberately severed it, producing additional agony and walking difficulties.[16]

In a health care system dominated by corporate interests, unusual problems with the law of consent could arise as a result of surgeons wishing to obtain tissue or DNA samples for research, or to use experimental techniques or equipment, then making such actions a covert or explicit condition of patients obtaining access to treatment. Another problem situation could be when a surgeon sustains a needle-stick and blood is taken without consent from the anaesthetised patient to check for transmissible disease such as HIV infection (generally because it is inconvenient and often unproductive to wait for the patient to wake and then seek consent). What options does a subsequently woken patient have to actually refuse consent, when the sample was necessary (according to hospital guidelines) to minimise corporate liability and justify continuing private health insurance coverage?

Beyond the era of the market state, health lawyers and policy makers will make much more in such circumstances, of the fact that a patient who suffers trespass to his or her body also experiences violation of the human right to physical integrity. Depending on the circumstances, non-consensual surgical invasion (or institutional guidelines and market state laws permitting such) will also be more uniformly recognised as breaching a patient's international human right to life, or the prohibition of cruel, unusual or degrading treatment.

Most importantly, Article 7 of the *ICCPR*, which requires 'free consent' before medical treatment or experimentation, will be more emphasised in such contexts. States are likely to provide increasing amounts of information on this proviso in their reports to the relevant UN committee. Some may regard it as creating obligations upon signatories only insofar as a state is responsible for the medical or scientific experimentation concerned. Increasingly, however, *ICCPR* Article 7 may be interpreted as according a right to 'protection' from 'private' third parties such as doctors, or the corporations that control them. Judges using such an international human right to develop the law in this area will accept certain public interest exceptions. An example would be the principle necessitating protection of a minor from imminent death or major injury, or society from an infectious disease epidemic.

A valid consent to treatment generally will continue to require documentation that the patient understood the nature of the procedure proposed and agreed to it. Courts will similarly hold that parental consent to medical treatment must be exercised in the 'best interests of the child', any uncertainty being resolved judicially. Once the child can be documented to have reached a sufficient level of comprehension (a mature minor), his or her consent will be sufficient to satisfy the legal requirements.

Whether or not the patient had the requisite mental capacity to consent will remain a contentious threshold question concerning legal liability for breach of consent. As well as minors, mentally impaired persons, or others whose consciousness is temporarily compromised (such as sedated or comatose intensive care patients), will fall into this category. Due to the extreme vulnerability of such patients, the ethical principle of respect for patient autonomy will be reinforced, in this context, by specific legislative protections. This may particularly be so in relation to reproductive-related or major surgery likely to irrevocably impinge on what may be termed the patient's life narrative and sense of personal identity and integrity (for example, plastic surgery, sterilisation or organ donation). In these circumstances, legislation will generally require consent to be obtained from guardianship boards where all the moral, ethical, legal and international human rights issues involved can be carefully weighed.

Another area likely to remain contentious is whether patients need to consent as having understood and agreed to not just the physical nature of the procedure, but its purpose within the regulatory framework of details such as the professional or unprofessional motivation of the health professional, and his or her qualifications. Courts, for example, have held that medical consent is vitiated where a patient submits to sexual interference under the mistaken belief that it formed part of a *bona fide* medical or surgical procedure. Failure by a doctor to disclose his or her infection with a potential transmissible disease, or professional registration, for example, may be viewed by the courts as overturning a patient's legal consent to treatment. Whether a doctor's failure to disclose possession of shares or other financial inducements (for example in a relevant medical device or pharmaceutical or health management company) is recognised by courts as having the same consent-vitiating effect will be a major test of the extent to which the laws of consent can be relied upon to protect the interests of patients.

In the post-market state era, it should more uniformly be considered a *prima facie* breach of medical professionalism for the state to pass legislation requiring particular individuals to donate organs or become involved in scientific research as a condition of access to health services or essential medicines. Such protections will be particularly important for subjects involved in clinical trials in developing nations.

III. Informed consent: The fictions of democratic legitimacy and patient autonomy

§i. *Informed consent, consumer choice and corporate legitimacy*

Laws requiring disclosure of, and free consent to, material risk prior to medical treatment or experimentation ('informed consent') are closely related to the ethical principle requiring respect for patient autonomy. They are widely regarded as having their origins (albeit in a research context) in the *Nuremberg Code* enunciated in 1948 after the Nazi doctors' trial. The first common law statement of the doctrine of informed consent was by Justice Bray in *Salgo v Leland Stanford Jr University Board of Trustees* in 1957. This appears to have been an unattributed incorporation of ethical principles drafted by a law firm as part of an *amicus curiae* brief submitted on behalf of the American College of Surgeons.[17]

Globally, the laws of informed consent provide a good example of a type of social contract dialogue about the extent to which a regulatory system should support patient involvement in health care decision-making. German courts, for example, appear to support, as a general principle of law, the inverse relationship between degree of medical urgency to avoid serious injury and the extent of disclosure required.[18] The Irish Supreme Court has held that in elective surgery related to sexual capacity (vasectomy), even statistically rare risks (for example, orchalgia) need to be disclosed.[19] The Japanese Nagoya District Court has confirmed the wide degree of discretion given to a doctor to withhold information (a cancer diagnosis) before the patient's right to self-determination is infringed.[20] A US court has emphasised the legal fiduciary duty of doctors to fully disclose relevant financial conflicts of interest to a patient choosing whether or not to request or agree to a procedure.[21]

In the United States, informed consent is often regarded as premised on a constitutional right to self-determination; a similar concept is the basis of the doctrine in Japan.[22] In Australia, the principle is referred to as 'disclosure of material risk', and the High Court there has rejected its basis in any 'right to self determination' – that was considered more appropriate in relation to consent negativing assault and battery.[23] The German Federal Supreme Court (Bundesgerichsthof) has conceptually founded informed consent upon respect for the patient's 'freedom and dignity as a human being'.[24] The French Supreme Court (Cour de Cassation) has likewise given the doctrine a theoretical basis in 'respect for the human being'.[25] In South Africa, Australia and the United Kingdom, judicial decisions have found that the courts (not the profession or, presumably, its corporate managers) should be the ultimate arbiters of the standard of care in informed consent.[26]

In some jurisdictions, however, medical indemnity insurers have successfully lobbied governments that such 'liberal' informed consent laws were becoming a *de facto* 'no fault' compensation scheme (by lowering the threshold of liability). The solution lobbied for and accepted involved legislation that subsidised their (the insurers') costs, reinstituted the restrictive professional practice standard of care and otherwise made it difficult for injured patients to sue using the informed consent doctrine.

As we move beyond a fully privatised global health care system, what types of information will doctors about to perform a medical intervention, procedure or therapy consider themselves bound by fundamental professional responsibilities to disclose to a competent patient? Will such information include carefully collected data on that (private) hospital's or surgeon's success or failure rates for that operation?

Will such disclosure be prevented by commercial-in-confidence claims related to patents over medical processes? In what detail will surgeons and physicians have to reveal any conflicts of interest implicit in their having received corporate gifts, or having shares in medical equipment or pharmaceutical companies? Will doctors merely have to present to a consumer what they, or their specialist college or company lawyers, consider the reasonably likely risks, without needing to discuss particular patient concerns? Without such information, how can patients still be sure that medical professionals are being loyal to relief of their suffering, rather than to the interests of their corporate employers or sponsors?

In the era of the market state, corporate health care managers have seen advantages in promoting informed consent as a single discrete event, like signing a contract. If so (they reasoned), why should not 'consumers' be at liberty to trade some informed consent rights for rapid movement up surgical waiting lists, a surgeon of their choice or even reduced out-of-pocket costs? In such circumstances, a legal duty of employee physicians to disclose in informed consent discussions that patient refusal to consent will not prejudice minimum ongoing care could create tension with health care employee contractual obligations.

Likewise, corporate health care managers have been unlikely to agree to legal obligations that their medical employees should disclose their operative success or failure, or post-operative complication rates, malpractice judgments and settled claims, medical board disciplinary actions, publication history, qualifications and honours. Surely to do so would put them at a business disadvantage against competitors? Consent forms have become quasi-contractual devices for limiting institutional and individual professional liability. The legal rules of informed consent remain a system of 'paper compliance' in which 'consumers' trade responsibilities in conformity with a judicial 'fairytale' of free will which is increasingly becoming a mere public relations exercise.

In the era of the market state, manufacturers of drugs have often found it convenient to lobby for a legal standard allowing them to prove (in the event of adverse drug reaction) that they defer to and had previously informed the relevant patient's doctor of the potential dangers – by, for example, package inserts, recommendations for prior genetic testing ('pharmacogenomics'), physician's desk references, and/or letters and information from drug 'reps'. Health care corporations, while desiring to advertise directly to patients, likewise could readily seek to shield themselves behind a 'learned intermediary'. Direct-to-consumer pharmaceutical advertising, despite pressuring clinicians into decisions that have often had a stronger marketing than evidence base, have made it clear that responsibility for prescriptions rests with the physician. Lawyers for health care corporations have been likely to claim that causation, in such instances, should be decided on the basis of complex 'but for' and 'loss of a chance' doctrines predicated on statistical probabilities, but not requiring empirical evidence.

In the post-market state age, however, health care product manufacturers will be less likely to succeed with arguments against causation of compensable damage being determined through judicial considerations of common sense, weighing empirical evidence and coherence between legal principles and foundational social and professional virtues. Neither will such corporate legal representatives so successfully maintain the case for an 'objective' test assessing reasonable probability that the patient/consumer had been fully informed of risks, simply because it was less likely to lead to liability than a 'subjective' test involving proof of actual disclosure.[27]

In the post-market state era, incorporation of legal rules about informed consent into an 'integrated' professional regulatory system will emphasise their deterrent role and encourage reforms (both legislative and judicial) seeking to shape such rules after broad and accurate research about their outcomes, in terms of equity in compensation, efficiency of process and improvement in public health. Improving the process of hearing and recording expert testimony about reasonably likely material medical risk will increase coherence between medical professional regulation and foundational social and professional virtues.

Generally acknowledged exceptions to the duty to disclose material risks prior to medical treatment or experimentation ('informed consent') will continue to be supported, but with greater vigilance about ways in which they may be covertly expanded to restrict patient protections. Two of the most significant are when a health professional has reasonable evidence that the disclosure would cause imminent and substantial harm (not mere anxiety) to this particular patient ('therapeutic privilege'), and when the context represents an emergency ('necessity').

Such exceptions will not allow health professionals during informed consent discussions to withhold information about therapeutically valuable pharmaceutical treatment alternatives merely because they consider patients likely to be distressed about their inability to afford them.[28] Instead, the influence of an 'integrated' professional regulatory system would be more likely to galvanise increasing numbers of health professionals to ensure that the price-setting mechanisms of pharmaceutical multinationals are fair and accountable. Necessity, similarly, will be less likely to be accepted as a convenient reason for assuming informed consent by all Emergency Departments of Intensive Care patients, regardless of their individual competence to decide.

To support foundational social and professional virtues in this setting, judges will resist pressures to restrict causes of action based on lack of informed consent. It would arguably be coherent for the law to provide a defence to a claim based on lack of informed consent if it is established that the patient would have gone ahead with the procedure or treatment anyway, regardless of what material risk information was or wasn't provided. Such a rule, however, may unfairly discriminate against poor patients with little choice about access to health care services, and may create an incentive for the laws of informed consent to be manipulated by corporate managers seeking to slough off responsibility under a 'consumer choice–consumer responsibility' model.

Under an 'integrated' system of medical professional regulation, an 'informed consent' discussion by a health professional will be required to comply with a broader range of ethical guidelines and international human rights standards, as well as law. This may involve an expected disclosure, for example, of all alternatives, benefits and discomforts, relevant test results, recent relevant adverse events, the patient's capacity to ask for a second opinion and the reasonably likely risks (as well as those particular or important to that patient) associated with use of specific drugs, equipment and procedures.

On the other hand, doctors working in the post-market state era may still feel they are being responsive to foundational professional virtues and principles if they do not disclose what they perceive to be the full hand of terrifying information when the patient is virtually a prisoner of the hospital system with little effective option but to proceed. Most patients, they would claim, have sufficient trust in their doctors to not wish to be disturbed by such information. Others may rely on patients' differing cultural approaches to medical authority to justify non-disclosure. Some will highlight systemic institutional problems such as lack of time, or inappropriate circumstances, facilities and remuneration. They could regard over-enthusiastic application of the autonomy principle through informed consent as promoting a consumer-choice model which could create difficulties in areas such as prenatal genetic testing (readily facilitating terminations of pregnancy or pre-implantation sex selection for idiosyncratic reasons), plastic surgery and elective surgery generally. Such a model may encourage doctors' responsibility to warrant a particular result, not just performance at the requisite level of skill and care.

The quality of informed consent discussion will become one clear measure of the values underpinning a system moving away from a fully privatised health care model. The argument presented here is that these are more likely to receive community support and facilitate public safety if systematically organised within an 'integrated' system of professional regulation where virtue is the currency of choice.

§ii. *Research and informed consent: Asking too much?*

In the age of the market state, consumers, their tissue and health care data, have been increasingly viewed as valuable low-cost resources for product research and development. Policies requiring consumer involvement in clinical trials of new medicines as a condition of private health insurance coverage, or promoting such participation as a viable alternative for consumers unable to afford expensive innovative medicines, were a logical outcome of market fundamentalist philosophies when applied to the health care sector. Corporate public relations 'spin' on such policies has promoted them as a way in which poor people can participate in the triumphs of innovative research over disease, their safety allegedly being protected by ethics committee scrutiny of research protocols and rigorous self-enforced industry standards.

Corporate pressure to obtain routine permission from consumers to perform potentially lucrative scientific research on genetic samples has become a major problem in the area of informed consent laws. Organisations seeking to properly fulfil their informed consent obligations in relation to storage of genetic data have had to choose between hiring certified informed consent counsellors, on the one hand, and contractually or legislatively restricting the organisation's responsibilities, on the other.

People participating in an informed consent discussion as part of a medical research project, particularly if they are poorly educated, or have language and/or cultural barriers to understanding, can often confuse a scientific investigator with a clinical doctor. They frequently fail to appreciate their statistical chance of only taking a placebo pharmaceutical, something that has no expected therapeutic effect.

Most patients will initially express much good will and altruism towards clinical trials ostensibly organised to discover 'truth' by randomisation, 'blinding' patient and doctor, using placebos, or by enhancing statistical 'power' through a large sample size. In doing this they are naturally responding positively to a system's emphasis on virtue, a psychological fact that underpins the 'integrated' professional regulatory system presented here. Many will also assume that they will be protected by the uniform application of research ethics principles such as those in the *Nuremberg Declaration*, which require that in the face of any conflict with such values, the interests of the individual research subject were to prevail.

Such social capital began to erode once potential research subjects, assuming their mantle as 'consumers', wished to be properly paid for their involvement and learnt of the extent to which the design, conduct and publication of such research was skewed by its corporate engineers away from objective scientific truth and towards outcomes favourable to the marketing of new pharmaceuticals and health care products. Similarly unsettling has been increased public knowledge that research trials conducted with a placebo arm were more inexpensive and more likely to produce favourable clinical results, without the risk of supporting a competitor's product.

Many patients/consumers found it similarly disturbing to learn how researchers attempted to sustain the myth of placebo analgesia, just as other privately 'hired' scientists had backed the myths that smoking did not cause cancer, or was not addictive and that global warming was merely a seasonal pattern or relatively benign climate change. During the World Medical Association's revisions of the global statement of medical research ethics known as the *Declaration of Helsinki*, for example, pharmaceutical company representatives and apologists argued that placebo-controlled trials should continue to be permitted where control patients were unlikely to die, become disabled or suffer serious harm.

Health professionals realised that disclosing the possibility of placebo randomisation in such circumstances might undermine the precise reason why many people without health insurance would grant their consent to participation in the relevant clinical trial. Many patients with HIV/AIDs, for example, were only able to gain access to expensive new drugs through participating in 'cutting edge' investigations of new therapies. For them, and sometimes their physicians, violating research protocols (by having their trial drug secretly analysed to see if it was placebo, for instance) became a form of conscientious non-compliance necessary to counterbalance a system that seemed out of tune with foundational virtues and principles.

In the post-market state era, placebo analgesia will increasingly be presumptively regarded as in breach of fundamental social and professional virtues and principles, including a state's absolute international human rights obligation not to inflict, and to take positive action to prevent, cruel and unusual treatment.

As global inequities in resource distribution are more rationally addressed by regulatory systems, people volunteering to be involved in medical research will be less likely to come primarily from impoverished, poorly educated populations with limited or no access to health care. Doctors involved in such research trials will be less likely to be restricted by protocols and employment contracts, and/or by corporate gifts and funding obligations, from openly discussing with patients their hunches or beliefs about what treatment would be most efficacious and whether or not a particular person should be in a placebo control group. Promises that patients will benefit from the research will be more consistently and genuinely honoured.

Also, an 'integrated' professional regulatory system will be rigorous in its requirement that clinical trials be based on an ethical principle of evidentiary/theoretical, or clinical, equipoise. This means that a precondition for their commencement will more uniformly be the absence of a clear consensus amongst the medical profession in relation to the alternative treatments being studied.

Finally, in the post-market state era, standards of medical professionalism will more strongly emphasise Article 7 of the *ICCPR*: 'No one shall be subjected without his free consent to medical or scientific treatment.' It is difficult to imagine how any such consent could be genuinely 'free' unless it is based upon an understanding of adequately disclosed material medical risk. Further, if legal principles and rules related to informed consent before medical research are widely regarded as part of international human rights law, they could more readily recirculate to assist in the evolution of a more coherent professional regulatory regime in domestic legal jurisdictions throughout the world. Such an approach emphasises human rights developing not in a legalistic way from consent of sovereign states, but as the outcome of a global community of principle that is also renegotiating a social contract about global health care and professionalism.

§iii. Systems error and 'consent' forms

Classical literary tragedies tell of protagonists who make a single wrong decision (*hamartia*), particularly as the result of an overarching fate (or influence of a grand system), and then suffer a pitiable reversal of fortune, heralded by discovery and recognitions. Modern directors of Shakespeare's tragedies have sought to make explicit this linkage between man's self-recollection and system-induced error. Imre Csiszar, for example, set *King Lear* in a decaying factory, Robert Sturua's 1987 *Lear* in Tbilisi ended with a simulated nuclear explosion, and Peter Brooks, following Jan Kott, interpreted Lear's predicament as similar to that created by arbitrary human rights violations in a police state.[29]

Beyond the era of the market state, health professional regulation will be more likely to systematically incorporate well-accepted insights from research in areas such as quality assurance in product manufacture and international aviation. Chief amongst these is that safety is not best ensured by attributing moral blame and legal culpability to individuals. Rather, it is necessary to examine deficiencies in the relevant institutional system.

Ninety per cent of aviation, industrial and anaesthetic accidents, for instance, have indeed ultimately been attributed, after routine post-adverse outcome and 'near miss' incident investigation, in some measure to human error.[30] Yet such error has been proven to arise predominantly through problems related to, for example, training, supervision, access to, and servicing of, equipment and maintaining rosters with sensible working hour requirements. Efforts have been made to introduce this notion, often in the guise of continuous quality improvement, generally into the health system. Yet in the age of the market state, this effort has never become widespread, uniform or effective, chiefly because of its perceived dissonance with corporate profit-making objectives both in health care management and in the privatised adversarial legal system that runs the fault-based compensation system for medical error.

In the post-market state era, however, such systems-based approaches to investigating and compensating medical error will become routine. The consent form is likely to play an important role in this process. Claims from the private health insurance industry that team-based professionalism, uniformly and consistently emphasising evidence-based medicine, has replaced the 'heroic' doctor model will be more carefully scrutinised in search of the industry's underlying policy objectives. Such a 'replacement', for example, could subtly denigrate the role of individual conscience in clinical decision-making, and so would have a problematic place in an 'integrated' professional regulatory system.

In an 'integrated' professional regulatory system, the legal rules of informed consent will be supported by much broader range of health professionals (including health corporate managers and policy-makers) as necessarily involving serial discussions and a genuine 'getting to know' between doctor and patient. Good data will become available about informed consent in practice. These empirical studies will no longer suffer from major conceptual and methodological flaws, including lack of adequate sample size and failure to investigate what was actually said in each case between doctor and patient. These factors may even see the term 'doctor–patient relationship' gradually replaced by the more accurate descriptor 'health system–patient relationship.'

In this context, consent forms will become a mechanism for ensuring that the majority of informed consent discussions prior to medical treatment or experimentation proceed along similar lines, with the same recognition of foundational professional virtues and principles.

The signing of a consent form prior to major surgery is already a standardised ritual throughout the medical world. Such instruments stand like surveyors' pegs, outlining the various territories of the professional and social contract about medicine: conscience, medical ethics, health law and international human rights. They are perhaps the one point at which the ideals and principles of medical professionalism can be made consistently and coherently relevant to the majority of individual patients and doctors.

Beyond the era of the market state, the medical profession will coordinate with relevant NGOs in urging the United Nations to assist with drafting a multinational treaty on universal health care and health technology regulation. Its obligations will include a commitment by state parties to developing, implementing and maintaining an International Model Medical Disclosure and Consent Form. It is only such a process that would be likely to successfully create adequate and uniform global standards for disclosure of financial conflicts of interest in informed consent discussions.

IV. The medical fiduciary: Can virtue be coerced?

Fiduciary obligations form a category of legal obligations, generally derived from the decisions of courts of equity and designed to protect people in presumptively vulnerable situations. The flexible content of the duties and remedies available through fiduciary law suggests it may have a critical role in medical professional regulation both in and beyond the age of the market state.

§i. Medical fiduciary duty as an antidote to corporate influence

The development of legal fiduciary duties is a story readily told as a judicial quest to fashion enforceable rules that promoted foundational professional virtues such as loyalty to the vulnerable and easily exploited.

In England, from the latter half of the 17th century, judges in Chancery searched for alternative, equitable remedies for breach of trust in relationships such as trustee and beneficiary, mortgagee and mortgagor, agent and principal, executor and beneficiary, company director and prospective shareholders, and between clients and bankers, share brokers and accountants. The Chancellor was often portrayed as the keeper of the King's conscience, protecting those who suffered, for example, as orphans and idiots, or as ruined suitors lacking monied might (a view sceptically explored by Dickens in *Bleak House*).

The doctor–patient relationship seemed to readily fall within these categories. If a patient alleged that a doctor had received a private benefit or gain from their relationship in circumstances creating a conflict of interest, the onus of proof was on the medical fiduciary to justify that gain. The patient only had to establish the appearance of disloyalty to justify a legal claim for breach of fiduciary duty. The onus of proving innocence was then on the doctor.

Judges in jurisdictions more likely to experience the relevant conflicts of interest created in a privatised health care system (such as the United States) have appeared more willing to impose a legal fiduciary duty on health professionals.[31] In Australia, where much health care still operates on a universal taxpayer-funded basis, judges from that nation's superior court have not seen a need to characterise the doctor–patient relationship as being comprehensively covered by legal rules of fiduciary responsibility.[32] They have emphasised instead that the primary legal duty of the doctor is to exercise reasonable care and skill in the provision of advice and treatment. It is not to act 'on behalf of' a patient, with 'undivided' or 'uncompromising' loyalty so as to avoid any conflict of interest whatsoever, or to warrant that treatment will be successful. There are, the court has held, only fiduciary 'elements' (or 'principles') in the relationship. These have evolved from the sensitive and intimate nature of patient reliance, the patient's need for bodily exposure, to divulge confidential information, and his or her presumed inability to fully protect personal economic interests.

These restricted 'fiduciary elements' have been expressed as legal rules requiring that doctors keep patient information confidential, receive no more than proper remuneration and do not procure gifts, nor sexually intimidate or abuse patients. The Court has been careful to leave open the capacity of the fiduciary concept to 'monitor the abuse of loyalty reposed in the medical practitioner by a patient', particularly where the doctor has obtained a commercial or financial benefit or gain from the patient beyond the agreed fee.

On one particularly idealistic view, beyond the age of the market state the medical professional will be perceived by regulators not just as the abstract 'reasonable man' of the common law. Instead, he or she will be viewed as a moral type, a mythical judicial 'everyman', protecting persons with unequal bargaining power who have reposed trust or confidence in him or her and thus become reliant, dependent or vulnerable in a professional context.

The fiduciary relationship, on this interpretation, may be placed atop a three-tiered hierarchy of fundamental equitable principles – above unconscionability and good faith – that is designed to regulate conduct in voluntary or consensual non-familial relationships. These three concepts can be reconceptualised as an ascending progression from permissible degrees of selfish to selfless professional behaviour.

Expanding the law of fiduciary obligations could include, for example, an obligation to promptly inform patients of adverse events or conflicts of interest concerning their treatment. Its application to health care corporate executives will be a valuable, but revolutionary development that balances their fiduciary obligations to maximise shareholder profits.

§ii. *Utmost loyalty in a disloyal system*

A major conceptual difficulty, however, will arise within an 'integrated' regulatory system when proposals are made to use legal fiduciary rules to enforce foundational professional virtues and principles. This problem is that virtue, necessarily arising from freedom to choose to consistently implement universally applicable principles in the face of obstacles, recedes before compulsion. It is a basic tenet of virtue theory, in other words, that regardless of the extent to which an act may be readily characterised as socially valuable, to develop virtue it must be a part of a series of reasoned acts that arise from a sense of duty (not from accident or coercion).

Judicial creation of the fully 'fiduciary' physician thus represents an extremely legalistic approach to regulation of medical professionalism. Like the canonical literary character Don Quixote, a doctor so rule-bound easily becomes a 'straw man' to be mocked and persecuted. This is because the requirement for such strongly obligatory legal armour and insignia may be viewed as an acknowledgment of the probable hollowness of his or her own personal commitment to professional ideals.

Indeed, in judicial decisions which proposed a fully fiduciary doctor–patient relationship, the language of virtue appeared to be incorporated in legal rules. At best this could represent a symbolic judicial encouragement to virtue, an appreciation that legal doctrine displaying words such as 'trust', 'confidence', 'influence', 'abuse of power', 'reliance', 'inequality' and 'vulnerability', as well as 'loyalty', as technical legal terms was likely to enhance coherence reasoning in an 'integrated' professional regulatory system. At worst, however, it constituted a judicial normative 'takeover', a depreciation of the synergistic role of virtue ethics in medical professional regulation. Such a legalistic approach to medical professionalism may promote a focus on the minimal standards required for avoidance of punishment and a diminution in motivation to rise in action beyond them.

So using fiduciary law to legally enforce professional virtues that are likely to be eroded by corporate influence over health care may become a two-edged sword. Fiduciary legal compulsion, for example, upon doctors to commence and continue expensive but 'futile' treatment, regardless of the needs of competing patients, would be consistent with the legalistic model of fiduciary rules covering the doctor–patient relationship. It could readily conflict, however, with fundamental virtues and principles of medical professionalism and the encouragement to make decisions using coherence reasoning, rather than simple, uncritical obedience to formal health law alone.

Beyond the age of the market state, legal fiduciary rules will continue to police important areas of clinical practice where patients are at high risk of exploitation due to criminal law's lack of an adequate deterrent function. They will threaten appropriately harsh sanctions against sexual impropriety by health professionals (regardless of the latters' defences to criminal charges of assault and battery, based on the supposed consensual nature of such interaction). They also may prevent managed care corporations, their employee clinicians or managers seeking, for example, to use surgical operation and research consent forms in attempts to contractually limit tortious or contractual liability to patients.[33]

Doctors compromising patient care by accepting pharmaceutical company 'kickbacks', lavish gifts, self-dispensing drugs or medical equipment, may also be deterred or punished by fiduciary legal rules. So may physicians, or health care corporate executives, who allow corporations to restrict length of hospital stay and/or deny marginal or expensive treatments, investigations or referrals.[34] These consequences will follow from the relationship between corporate health care executive or manager and patient (as well as shareholder) being characterised as fiduciary in nature.

An illustrative case study of the ongoing relevance of fiduciary law to medical professional regulation is *Moore*'s case.[35] Moore was a patient whose blood, skin, bone marrow aspirate, spleen, sperm and other genetic material were removed by physicians in the course of his numerous visits to their medical centre. The reason initially involved treatment of the patient's hairy cell leukaemia, but increasingly became dominated by his doctors' interest in potentially lucrative research involving recombinant DNA techniques. The physicians managed to develop a cell line from the patient's T-lymphocytes which they patented and called the 'Mo line'. They then negotiated contracts for its commercial development, receiving US$1.7 million and shares from the companies Genetics Institute and Sandoz. The Supreme Court of California held that the legal fiduciary duties of the relevant doctors involved a responsibility to disclose 'all information material to the patient's decision' to undergo treatment, including financial conflicts of interest.

Finally, in the age beyond the market state, open disclosure policies, in the past resisted by health care institutions reluctant to admit the occurrence of major adverse events, may be facilitated (in an 'integrated' professional regulatory system) by non-legal regulatory strategies such as 'open disclosure mentors', as well as by judicial categorisation of such conduct as part of a health professional's fiduciary duty.

V. Contract: Should vulnerable patients contractually bargain?

It has been argued here that the ideal preconditions for a renegotiated global social contract concerning medical professionalism and leadership include one particular consensual recognition by those who govern society at domestic and international levels. This is that human suffering, though inevitable, should be relieved both with the expression of, and in order to promote, individual and collective virtues such as therapeutic loyalty, justice and respect for human dignity.

These fundamental beliefs do not sit easily alongside the policy position, dominant in nations such as the United States and influential bodies such as the WTO, that global health services should be allocated chiefly through a variety of individual contractual bargains that give documentary form to the operation of largely unrestrained market forces. Yet in some jurisdictions supporting universalist health care policies, France in particular, civil code requirements have resulted in contract (rather than the common law of non-contractual wrongs based on reasonable foreseeability) receiving greater emphasis as a form of medical professional regulation.

This section examines the role that the law of contract might play in regulation of medical professionalism beyond the age of the market state.

§i. *The contract as a dominant mode of doctor–patient relations*

The contractual approach to regulating rather than preventing private profit in areas such as medical professionalism may have begun with the London physician Bernard Mandeville's book *Fable of the Bees* (1705). This work, with its emphasis on the social value of self-interest ('Vice is beneficial found, when 'tis by justice lopped and bound'), stimulated the free enterprise philosophy of Adam Smith – and, no doubt, of many legislators and common law judges. In a fully privatised global health care system, the primary contracts involved are likely to be between the doctor and his or her employing corporation. Their purpose, the maximisation of corporate and professional private financial gain, has the potential to cut across traditional professional service obligations to patients.

If the doctor–patient relationship is viewed primarily as a contractual bargain, a doctor's, or health care institution's, promise to confer benefit by relieving suffering theoretically requires some tangible consideration as fair exchange and may justify a health care 'consumer's' claim of detrimental reliance on that 'provider's' promise, if it is not fulfilled. Alternatively, the capacity for health care consumers to potentially contract away their rights and protections in this situation could be part of a broader free market ideology indicating the state's tolerance of free will and choice in arrangements between citizens and private corporations about services and property.

Judges in the United Kingdom have held that doctors impliedly contract with their patients to act at all times in the best interests of the patient.[36] The High Court of Australia has referred to a doctor's general contractual duty to 'exercise reasonable care and skill in the provision of professional advice and treatment'.[37] In France the physician, though generally held to owe a contractual duty to exercise reasonable care and skill (*obligation de moyens*), also has a duty to achieve a specific result (*obligation de résultat*), not only where such is explicitly warranted, but also where the medical activity is to a greater extent under his or her full control.[38]

One established implied contractual duty that is likely to conflict with corporate health care interests is a doctor's obligation to keep the patient's information confidential. A similar contractual duty requires a doctor to disclose information (but not necessarily the actual medical record) to the patient when the request is reasonable and refusal would prejudice the patient's health. The doctor is generally held by property law to own the material upon which the professional information is recorded, but it is unclear whether the same is true of the narrative itself.

The common conceptual thread to these legalistic interpretations of medical professionalism is that they conceptualise the relationship between health care system and patient components as property and its 'actors' as autonomous individuals able to trade an enforceable promise, at arm's length, for adequate consideration. Such a model, of course, fits neatly within the 'consumer choice' approach to health care services promoted by corporate interests, with its implicit transfer of much responsibility to the purchaser and capacity for sellers to structure bargains so that they minimise liability.

Common law courts have shown a readiness to imply into any contract such general principles of law and terms of fact as are considered necessary to give it efficacy, or protect the legal rights of related, presumptively vulnerable, parties. A contract-based doctor–patient relationship could thus be viewed by an 'integrated' professional regulatory system as involving implied principles that recognise the patient's inequality of knowledge and thus bargaining power.

In the age beyond the market state, universal health care schemes financed by taxpayers could similarly be regarded as presumptively altering the individual contractual premises of promise and reciprocal consideration between health systems and patients in favour of greater coherence with foundational professional and social virtues as expressed in a global social contract.

§ii. Bargaining the body and 'gag' clauses

Increased 'contractualisation' of medical professional regulation, however, may favour the interests of patients if the law grants them the capacity to trade a property interest in their genetic material. Property in one's own body is held by many theorists to be essential for individual protection, self-realisation and self-identity. Persons may be legally viewed as having a right to possession and use of their DNA, which leads to a correlative duty in others to avoid interference.

It may thus be very important, if we are to move beyond the value and health outcome problems implicit in a fully privatised global health care system, for patients to be able to assert under law a privilege to refuse a request for a genetic sample, and a power (creating correlative liability) to alienate it through donation to a sperm bank or DNA data bank. Likewise significant will be patients' contractual immunity (creating correlative disability) from genetic expropriation, even if necessary to save another's life (as with reluctant bone marrow donors). In the latter circumstance, other elements of the 'integrated' professional regulatory system would encourage and facilitate altruism. Similarly, granting an individual's genetic material (such as frozen embryos or sperm) and genetic information legal status as a type of *sui generis* quasi-property that can be traded could encourage greater equity and justice in negotiations between patients and health care corporations.

Shakespeare's *Merchant of Venice* provides interesting reflections in this context. The story of the way Shylock's contract making a pound of human flesh surety for a debt becomes nullified by the 'gentle rain' of equity provides a particularly apposite analogy for problems with 'commodifying' the human body, as expressed in areas such as surrogacy, organ donation from adults, use of 'made-to-measure' cloned organs, and ownership of frozen embryos or reproductive tissue. The director Ellis Rabb made this point about the intersection of business and broader equitable interest in the human body by making Shakespeare's Belmont a luxury yacht anchored in a lagoon; and Peter Zadek portrayed Shylock as a 1980s corporate raider.[39]

In *Moore*'s case (where doctors patented a cell line from a patient's tissue sample without prior consent), some judges, though aware of the injustice of allowing the health professionals involved to retain the 'fruits' of their disloyalty, also had concerns about the 'effect on human dignity of laws permitting a marketplace in human body parts'.[40] The majority ultimately refused to accept that legal principles respecting human privacy and dignity allowed individual human beings to profit from their own body. If this means the court decided that corporate interests can so profit (perhaps because they are presumed to lack a necessary connection with such foundational social virtues), then the case would be unlikely to be followed by a post-market state judiciary working within an 'integrated' professional regulatory system.

In the post-market state era, protection of the human genome from financial exploitation will increasingly be recognised as an established international bioethical, human rights and legal norm.[41] A major issue then may be whether medical professionalism should allow a patient to contractually bargain his or her capacity to suffer (for the purposes of scientific experimentation) for private gain – for an honorarium, salary, fee or at the behest of a third party. Can such a right be regarded as consistent with fundamental social and professional virtues and principles?

A related issue concerns contracts that doctors employed by managed care corporations may have signed. These can include clauses permitting 'no-cause' non-renewal of employment, linking salary with cost of care, restricting leave allowances and requiring fixed amounts of overtime. Doctors may also be 'gagged' by the same workplace agreement from disclosing to patients useful health services not covered by the authorised plan. They could similarly be contractually required to limit the ordering of tests, referrals, the utilisation of facilities, the duration of hospital admissions and number of procedures, or possibly even the full discussion of clinical cases with physicians 'owned' by other companies.

The sanction of loss of employment creates unprecedented corporate negotiating leverage concerning such contractual terms in a fully privatised health care system where many doctors have debts equivalent to a house mortgage on graduation, little option but to accept increased working hours with decreased entitlements and greater uncertainty about long-term job prospects.

Public interest exceptions to such contracts will need to be legally created to ensure that patients have a reasonable idea that a treatment option is being withheld and thus can recognise the need for a second opinion.

VI. Confidentiality and privilege: Protecting trust and loyalty

An 'integrated' system of regulating medical professionalism in the post-market state age will need to ensure that its principles and rules support a 'space' where patient trust and physician loyalty to the relief of suffering can flourish under the protection and respect of government. The legal doctrines of confidentiality and privilege of doctor–patient communications are likely to be particularly relevant in this context.

§i. Trading in secrets and data linkage

Colleagues, patients and the community as a whole regard a doctor's commitment to confidentiality as a sentinel measure of his or her professionalism. In 1996 the French *Tribunal de Grande Instance* suspended distribution of a book by President Mitterand's former doctor entitled *The Great Secret*. The work was alleged to breach ethical principles and legal rules requiring respect for the confidentiality of patient information. A different approach was taken in England in 1965 when a biography of Churchill was posthumously published by his physician, Lord Moran. Moran was shunned at his club and disapproving letters were written about him in professional journals. The British Medical Association used the controversy to affirm its stance on the centrality to medical professionalism of the ethical principle (derived originally from the *Hippocratic Oath*) that confidentiality continues after the death of the patient.

Another example highlights the risks to patients if doctors view confidential information obtained professionally as a source of personal profit. In 2003, a director of radiation oncology at the US Staten Island University Hospital was censured, reprimanded and fined $5000 for giving interviews to the press while treating the dying Beatle George Harrison. The doctor was alleged to have breached ethical and legal obligations to respect confidentiality by revealing in public, without the consent of the patient, personally identifiable information obtained in a professional capacity. He told reporters that Harrison, composer of the evocative songs *All Things Must Pass, My Sweet Lord, The Inner Light, Give Me Love (Give me Peace on Earth), Isn't it a Pity* and *Within You and Without You*, 'wasn't afraid of death and was writing songs to the end'. He also claimed Harrison had played for him and had given his son a guitar lesson. Whilst such actions hardly seem in the highest range of reprehensible professional conduct, the patient's reaction, and that of his relatives, indicate the seriousness attached to the expectation of confidentiality. Harrison's family sued the doctor for $10 million, claiming that this doctor had coerced this frail mystic remnant of the 'fab four' into autographing his son's guitar and signing autographs for his daughters, then given an interview to the *National Enquirer* to increase the value of this memorabilia.

A foundational ethical obligation to keep a patient's information confidential flows rationally from the vulnerability and need to trust implicit in the fundamental circumstances of doctor–patient relations. It may also be implied from the complementary ethical principles of beneficence and, in particular, respect for patient autonomy. It appears explicitly not only in the *Hippocratic Oath* and its modern reformulations, but in all domestic and international codes of medical ethics.

Breach of confidentiality is presumed to arise when a doctor releases information acquired in the professional relationship to a third party (outside the treating team) without the patient's permission. Such an action threatens proceedings for professional misconduct, as well as a damages claim based on breach of fiduciary duty, implied contractual terms, or the tortious standard of care for negligence and defamation. In many jurisdictions – including France, Germany, Belgium, Switzerland, Poland, Austria, the Netherlands, Argentina and Japan – failure to protect patient confidentiality can constitute a criminal offence.

Legal rules protecting the confidentiality of patient information may be particularly valuable in a fully privatised health care system. They may stop such information being traded for the purposes of research, or otherwise for corporate profit, without the patient's agreement or recompense.

Within health care systems in and beyond the age of the market state, increasingly large numbers of persons, both known and unknown to any patient, physically (especially in hospitals) and via electronic communications systems, will have access to medical records. Their reasons for such access will variously relate to clinical work, corporate profit, quality assurance and scientific research. There is, in particular, much potential for corporate profit and minimisation of expenses in gaining access to communications between doctor and patient. A large multinational company that funds private health insurance for its employees, for example, will perceive advantages in discovering whether or not any of its staff has HIV/AIDS. If the person does, the company then has the option of pre-emptively terminating his or her employment and thus not being burdened by disputes over expensive private health insurance payouts.

In the era of the market state, patient confidentiality, insofar as it has been enforced by ethical and legal rules, has been frequently circumvented by health professionals, including corporate health care managers. Civil actions for its breach have been rare, though, because of the expense of involving lawyers (even a 'no win-no fee' basis includes considerable disbursement charges), the increasing problems with obtaining legal aid and the difficulty of proving the act in question, as well as any consequent damage.

In the era of the market state, exceptions to the legal rules of medical confidentiality and privilege have proliferated, some in the interest of society and others merely to the benefit of corporations. Codes of medical ethics or guidelines have required a health professional to disclose information relevant to the health of a third party, such as the HIV/AIDS status of a sexual partner. Legislation has imposed public health duties to report, for example, births and deaths, illegal ownership of guns, gun and knife wounds, contraction of notifiable diseases and child abuse. In the controversial Californian decision of *Tarasoff*, a psychologist at a university hospital was found liable for failing to breach medical confidentiality and warn a person previously unknown to him (not merely the police, whom he did tell), after one of his patients disclosed a real and immediate intention to kill that third person.[42]

Confidentiality of genetic information will be an increasingly difficult issue in this context. A court has held, for example, that the physician of a mother with hereditable medullary thyroid carcinoma was not required to breach confidentiality and inform a daughter who later suffered the same disease.[43] In another case, judges found that the doctor of a father with hereditary *polyposis coli* predisposing to bowel cancer should have breached confidentiality to warn a daughter who subsequently developed the same condition.[44]

Where a doctor has been employed to examine a health consumer by a third party (for instance a health insurance company, the military or a potential employer), the law has recognised that a prior contractual arrangement may alter legal obligations of confidentiality. In the era of the market state, legal exceptions permitting a doctor to disclose patient information relevant to potential commission of a serious crime may have also been manipulated to fit agendas related to the so-called war on terrorism.

In the post-market state age, information given in confidence by a patient is likely to be more widely recognised as immune from judicial discovery or subpoena, and doctors regarded as less readily compellable witnesses about their interactions with patients. In such instances there will be, in other words, a more established legal privilege protecting communications between patient and doctor. The doctor and patient in such circumstances will no longer have to rely upon the *de facto* privilege of judicial discretion.

Under 'integrated' professional regulation, the more substantial the interference with the ethical principle of respect for patient autonomy and the patient human right to privacy, the more a court may require by way of justification before it is satisfied that any decision to breach medical confidentiality is reasonable.[45]

Legal professional privilege, for example, may be granted to hospital mortality reviews or deliberations of clinical ethics committees, but not to situations where a physician is consulted chiefly to satisfy a third party requirement (for example, for insurance or worker's compensation purposes). This may be of great importance given the commercial interest of insurers and employers in the genetic information (such as genetic susceptibility to disease) that may have flowed from such examination.

In *Z v Finland*, for example, the European Court of Human Rights held that 'careful scrutiny' was required where 'intimate and sensitive' information (such as HIV/AIDS status) was set to be disclosed.[46] Courts will pay more uniform attention to human rights principles related to confidentiality – including 'compelling justification', 'pressing social need', 'proportionality' and 'proximity' concerning a doctor's ability to readily identify the victim, and a 'real and immediate' risk to the third party's life – that have been set out in decisions of the European Court of Human Rights concerning articles of the *European Convention on Human Rights*.[47]

Precepts of the *Universal Declaration of Human Rights*, such as the human right not to be subjected to 'arbitrary interference with privacy', to protection of the family, to freedom of thought and conscience and to seek, receive and impart information, are likely to become increasingly important in coherence reasoning concerning professional obligations to respect confidentiality.

VII. Criminal law: Abortion and euthanasia

§i. *Abortion: Conscientious objection and deontological imperatives*

When Dr Henry Morgentaler and other medical practitioners opened a clinic in Ontario (Canada) to perform abortions, they did so in the knowledge that they would be arrested. This act of civil disobedience resulted, as the doctors hoped, in a Supreme Court decision holding that substantial danger to the physical or mental health of a requesting mother provided a legal justification for abortion, particularly in the first trimester. Nonetheless, many doctors performing abortions were subsequently (and continue to be) subjected to acts of terror and violence by those advocating the fetal right to life. This section considers how the uneasy normative compromise on the issue of abortion is likely to fare in and beyond a fully privatised global health care system.

The legal systems of most developed nations have achieved a hard-fought compromise over medical involvement in termination of pregnancy (medically assisted abortion). This compromise makes abortion a statutory criminal offence if done without maternal consent, or after the point of viability (when the presumptively vulnerable fetus has the capacity for independent existence outside the womb). It renders such a procedure lawful, however, if it is requested voluntarily by the mother and is necessary to protect her from a serious and abnormal danger to her life or physical or mental health.

The successful balancing of normative concerns involved here is a good example of how an extremely contentious issue for medical professionalism may be incorporated by democratic processes into the fabric of a social contract. Part of this balancing involves regulatory recognition that many doctors and private health care corporations, particularly those endorsing Catholic religious principles, openly refuse to facilitate abortion because they believe in protecting the sanctity of fetal life, a moral principle they derive from both general theology and the *Hippocratic Oath*.[48]

Basic tenets of medical professionalism in this context require that patients seeking termination (even if approaching a doctor or health care organisation that will not endorse that procedure, on religious grounds) should not be abandoned by health professionals. Instead, they should be referred to practitioners holding an equally coherent (and often equally religious view) supporting a woman's moral, ethical and legal right to choose in these circumstances. For both groups of doctors, though, failing to treat the *results* of an abortion, or to assist a woman in a medical emergency related to an abortion, would undoubtedly contradict the basic principles of medical professionalism.

Prenatal screening programs and tests (more likely to be readily available to the privately insured) that detect untreatable fetal disorders chiefly in order to give parents the option of abortion are logical extensions of the 'consumer choice' model of health care dominant under market state health care systems. Such investigations can place pressure on doctors loyal to the relief of patient suffering to perform acts of civil disobedience or conscientious non-compliance, depending on whether their own consciences, in such circumstances, achieve a justifiable coherence of principle.

In the midst of such deliberations, medical professionals might consider two primary objections (based on principles derived from personal religious views, bioethics and international human rights) to the deliberate killing of a developing human embryo. The first presupposes and is derived from natural rights and those protectable interests the social contract grants to all human beings (contentiously including fetuses). The second does not depend upon or presume any particular rights, interests, or potential life narrative capacity in the fetus. Instead, it claims that abortion is wrong in principle because it disregards and insults the intrinsic value, the sacred character, of human life at any stage or form.[49]

Medical professionals may equally consider the principle that a woman forced to give birth to a child she does not want suffers a deprivation of that liberty and capacity for autonomy and self-determination necessary to create a coherent life narrative. This is all the more true where the woman's decision to terminate the pregnancy factored in the origins of that condition in rape or incest, known serious fetal genetic abnormalities, or a fundamental lack of the economic and emotional support necessary to raise a child in a loving environment. An 'integrated' professional regulatory system would be well placed to help health professionals realise that women in such circumstances often experience social and professional abandonment and lack of understanding which makes them even more vulnerable to exploitation and neglect.

Such a regulatory system is also likely to assist health professionals to understand that in many developing countries where abortion remains illegal, maternal choice is additionally silenced by policies promoting illiteracy, poverty, censorship of information, discriminatory social taboos and poor statistical records, as well as apathy and corruption amongst public health officials.

Health professionals trained and working within an 'integrated' system of professional regulation will be more able to calibrate decisions such as that in *Rust v Sullivan*[50] against contrary norms of medical ethics and international human rights. In that case, the US Supreme Court upheld federal regulations preventing doctors working in federally funded clinics from discussing abortion with patients. The majority judges reasoned that the women involved could get such advice elsewhere. If a state's laws prohibit abortion, the practice will not cease, for a variety of personal maternal reasons which will require health professionals, should they choose to respect them, to engage, as they have in the past, in conscientious non-compliance.

In the era of the market state, some governments have refused foreign aid to agencies whose programs in developing nations facilitate safe medical abortion, despite having 'liberal' abortion laws in their own jurisdiction. As we move beyond this period, however, a broad range of health professionals will increasingly find such policy inconsistencies incoherent with foundational principles of medical ethics and international human rights.

Beyond the era of the market state, policy battles are likely to be fought over an alleged human right of procreative autonomy, arguably covering the capacity to reproduce with or without information about the genes potentially involved. Coherence reasoning within an 'integrated' professional regulatory system is best suited to decide whether such a right, if made part of health law, should protect parents from denial of insurance coverage for failing to genetically test their fetus, or for refusing to treat any major detected abnormality by *in utero* somatic gene therapy.

§ii. *Should cost determine if end of life care is futile?*

This section considers how medical professionalism and leadership should operate in relation to end of life decisions as we move beyond a fully privatised global health care system. As the population continues to age in developed nations, more elderly 'ex-consumers' will be seeking places in private nursing homes where the regular attendance of doctors is becoming more problematic. Many will wish to control the extent of medical interventions in their final illnesses, both for reasons of dignity and because of the cost to themselves and their family.

In *Metamorphosis*, Franz Kafka describes a person waking from uneasy dreams to find himself transformed into a big cockroach. *Metamorphosis* is likely to resonate with the increasing numbers of people in the developed world who, after accident or illness, regain consciousness to find themselves as a health care 'consumer' in a privatised Intensive Care Unit.

Their body is now bedridden, immobilised and sprouting therapeutic and monitoring lines and wires. They are mostly voiceless because of an endotracheal tube through which a machine intermittently supplies gas under positive pressure to help expand and oxygenate their lungs. Infusions of drugs support their heart and blood pressure, also keeping pain and anxiety suppressed, though at the expense of clouding consciousness. They receive tasteless nutrition through a central venous line. Their urine drains without effort via a catheter. They are washed by nurses, regularly 'examined' and spoken about by doctors, as if they are some intellectual puzzle involving physiological and biochemical numbers. The staff records and protocols of this privatised health care system prefer to call them 'consumers' ... a designation whose callous insincerity in such tragic circumstances exposes the normative weaknesses of market fundamentalism when applied to health care.

Kafka's story depicts how difficult it is for other people to feel empathy for such a creature. To assist such a patient/consumer's recovery, relatives often place photographs of the person, in normal surroundings, around the hospital bed. They talk to a comatose patient about the small events of the day and hold his or her hand, as if awareness were present. When the clinical notes (as they mostly do not) include references to the patient's favourite music, books or activities, dreams and hopes, staff are more motivated, as they have a stronger intuitive conviction about relieving this patient's suffering.

One of the most poignant ethical moments for a health professional in intensive care may involve a determination of what capacity for good, or quality of life, or opportunity to create a subjectively meaningful and coherent life narrative, this course of treatment is likely to permit a patient. The law provides that treatment proven to offer no prospect of return to a meaningful quality of life may be termed technically 'futile' and may be withdrawn or withheld.

The appraisal of clinical 'futility' may be done objectively, under the English 'best interests' test,[51] or subjectively, according to the North American 'substituted judgment', which emphasises evidence of the patient's wishes from relatives, close friends or the existence of an advance treatment directive (living will), health care power of attorney or guardianship order.[52] A legalistic approach to protecting the interests of patients could involve suggesting that all such withdrawal and withholding of treatment decisions should be made by a court of law.

A position more in accord with an 'integrated' system of medical professional regulation, however, would be that a withdrawal or withholding of treatment decision is best made by consensus between treating doctors and family after repeated discussions attempting to reconcile the medical prognosis with knowledge of what the person would have recognised as a minimally acceptable quality of life. Involvement of a hospital's clinical ethics committee may be useful in circumstances where some or all relatives and doctors remain intractably in disagreement about such a decision. In each instance, the focus under 'integrated' professional regulation should be on maintaining coherence not only within the life narrative which has hitherto given that patient's life meaning, but also between the relevant principles of medical ethics, health law and international human rights.

In the *Bland* case, a UK House of Lords judicial decision concerning withdrawing and withholding treatment, Lord Hoffmann set out his reasons so that 'the decision of the court should be able to carry conviction with the ordinary person as being based not merely on legal precedent but also upon acceptable ethical values':

> In my view the choice which the law makes must reassure
> people that the courts do have full respect for life, but that they
> do not pursue the principle to the point at which it has become
> almost empty of any real content and when it involves the
> sacrifice of other important values such as human dignity and
> freedom of choice.[53]

In the era of the market state, such decision-making regularly has to also include factors such as a consumer's lack of private health insurance, or a relative scarcity of intensive care beds available for fully insured consumers. Imagine the distress for a family knowing that the intensive care treatment that may (or of course may not) save the life of their loved one will also possibly bankrupt them. Should such financial ruin as a consequence of accessing health care really be a matter of private 'consumer' choice and responsibility, of financial capacity to pay insurance premiums or obtain employment with health insurance coverage?

In the post-market state age, a medical professional considering withdrawal and withholding of medical treatment is likely to get positive institutional support for attempting to implement the following relevant principles reasonably derived from coherence reasoning applied to foundational professional and social virtues. First, respect for the doctor's primary professional role of relieving human suffering makes it *prima facie* wrong to shorten the life of a patient. Second, medical treatment nonetheless may be withheld or withdrawn where prolonging the life of a patient may exacerbate suffering, defined broadly to include consideration of coherence in a patient's life narrative.

Third, a competent patient is entitled to trust in medical respect for his or her will to go on living, although it may objectively appear that any related capacity to develop a coherent life narrative will be severely impaired. Fourth, it is morally, ethically and legally wrong to withdraw or withhold medical treatment where that process itself causes suffering. Fifth, it is similarly wrong to withdraw or withhold treatment to permit other patients to get access to a hospital bed, to reduce the cost of medical care, or to fulfil other political or corporate purposes of the state.

In the post-market state age, courts (like the English House of Lords, in *Bland*) will be more willing and able to weigh the applicability of the human right of sanctity of life by reference to its presence in the *ECHR* and the *ICCPR*. This will be so even if neither of those international human rights instruments is formally recognised in that jurisdiction as relevant law under doctrines of conservative legal positivism.[54] In *Pretty's Case and Application*, both the House of Lords and the European Court of Human Rights held that Article 8 of the *ECHR* protecting respect for private life applied to issues of quality of life in promoting human freedom and dignity for patients with terminal illness.[55]

In that age, health professionals will be more open and insightful in their critical analysis of policies promoting, as a means of facilitating 'consumer' choice, advance directives (statements of minimally acceptable quality of life), living wills or durable powers of attorney for health care. One of their chief concerns will be that the capacity of such instruments to reduce long-term costs of care should not take precedence over foundational virtues and principles of medical professionalism. Perhaps even more important will be the need to ensure that there is not even the appearance of such influence over no-cardiopulmonary resuscitation (no-CPR) orders for hospitalised patients. No-CPR orders are a type of advance directive which may facilitate patient autonomy and dignity in dying, while protecting doctors from liability once further treatment has been deemed clinically 'futile'.

In the age of the market state, advance directives purportedly perpetuating patient autonomy beyond the point of incapacity have been an attractive form of professional regulation from a legalistic, as well as a corporate managerial, perspective. They have generally been a written quasi-contractual document (though oral forms have also been permitted). This has facilitated external review of compliance in a manner with which lawyers are familiar. The common law in many jurisdictions has accepted them as overriding any legal duty of standard of care derived from the ethical principle of beneficence.[56] In the age of the market state, legislation has increasingly not only prescribed their form and mode of authorisation, but also encouraged their completion upon hospital admission.

In the post-market state era, however, the international human rights law perspective on advance directives is likely to be more influential in health system governance. This perspective views advance directives as enhancing self-determination and marking a boundary for the state's interest in respecting and protecting the sanctity of human life and patient freedom from degrading treatment. Advance directives, more carefully drafted, will continue to be frequently used by patients whose beliefs about treatment are likely to lead to conflict with those of a therapeutically loyal doctor (for instance, Jehovah's Witnesses wishing to refuse blood transfusions, and patients suffering from chronic debilitating illness who desire to 'pass away' with their human dignity respected).

§iii. Euthanasia and double effect in a for-profit setting

The story *It's Over Debbie*, published in the *Journal of the American Medical Association*, relates how an anonymous medical resident deliberately killed a 20-year-old woman who was terminally ill from ovarian cancer. He had never seen this patient before being paged by the nursing staff because of her difficulty in 'getting rest'. Although he observed that she had 'air hunger', this junior health professional did not auscultate the chest; neither did he examine a chest x-ray or a blood gas analysis. The woman said, 'Let's get this over with.' Without consulting the admitting physician, the trainee doctor drew up a large dose of morphine. He administered it intravenously until the patient stopped breathing.[57]

Some physicians saw the controversy following publication of this story as involving the 'very soul' of medicine – was its 'moral centre' collapsing? They asserted that fundamental moral and ethical principles repudiated direct and intentional killing by physicians.[58] Others stated that *It's Over Debbie* highlighted, as a matter of principle, how in clinical medicine, dogmatic adherence to absolutist moral or ethical principles should always be capable of being tempered by the spirit of virtues such as mercy. Modern medicine, they claimed, should not place the prolongation of death ahead of relief of individual patient suffering in a terminal illness.[59]

Euthanasia can be conceptualised as active (the physician's role being direct and primary) or passive (the doctor having a secondary role, as in physician-assisted suicide). It may be voluntary, involuntary (patient refuses), non-voluntary (patient incompetent), or a mix.

Questions of euthanasia or physician-assisted suicide occur more frequently amongst those terminally ill patients who believe that their suffering threatens to fundamentally undermine the virtue and coherence of their life narrative. Such persons commonly believe that their pain can be controlled by palliative care medicine, but their loss of human dignity can't. It is largely to regain this control, so that their end of life will be consistent with the narrative sense of integrity they perceive as characterising their whole life, that they approach doctors to seek assistance with dying.

Central to personal and professional narrative coherence here should be the foundational moral, ethical and international human rights principle requiring respect for the sanctity of human life. This regards all (post-birth) human life as being of equal value and makes it always wrong, regardless of the consequences, to intentionally kill a human being. The sanctity of life principle can be fed into moral syllogisms, or institutionally housed in a code of professional ethics and then applied to give practical guidance for clinical and health policy decisions. Legal rules prohibiting euthanasia may be viewed as contributing to an international community of principle (or even a global social contract renegotiation) particularly emphasised by medical professional institutions after the Nazi doctors' trial, that opposes totalitarian health policy 'tyrannies' such as those involved with pro-eugenics legislation.[60]

Yet in a society whose laws reflect principles derived from foundational virtues such as justice, fairness, liberty, respect for human dignity and loyalty to the relief of patient suffering, the state should respect the freedom of patients to make the critical decisions (as long as those decisions do not interfere with such freedoms in others) that shape their life narrative, their destiny and conscience, their conception of the meaning and value of human existence.[61]

In the age of the market state, however, disciples of market fundamentalism have frequently contended with religious acolytes interested in health policy over legislation permitting voluntary euthanasia. This has been true even if stringent conditions – such as the requirement for a proven conjunction of patient request, terminal illness, prior best-practice palliative care and the absence of any serious, treatable mental disorder – effectively reduced the risk of a recrudescence of non-voluntary euthanasia.[62]

Health care governance and regulatory systems generally recognise that withdrawal and withholding treatment is not euthanasia. This is chiefly because of the respective variations in clinical uncertainty of outcome. If the patient continues breathing after a decision of clinical futility and related withdrawal of the endotracheal tube and connection to the ventilator, for example, treatment must be continued. Similarly, the doctrine of 'double effect' also needs to be distinguished from euthanasia: it is professionally permissible to relieve pain, even up to the point of death. This clinical intention is best documented by use of a chart closely correlating incrementally increasing doses of intravenous analgesia with continuing pain symptoms.

Towards the conclusion of Kafka's story *Metamorphosis*, the once-human 'cockroach' describes how, having transformed into an insect, he becomes an outsider to his family. They talk about him as if he cannot listen, grow tired of the inconveniences his continued existence brings them and become oblivious to things that cause him suffering. A significant ethical risk with legal rules decriminalising euthanasia is not only abuse by the corporate managers seeking efficiencies, or physicians or family members who have allegiances that conflict with loyalty to the relief of patient suffering, but the fact that some terminally ill patients with a great respect for duty may see it as their responsibility to rid their loved ones of an unnecessary burden. My argument here is that the delicate process of balancing the individual and social moral, ethical and legal concerns involved with euthanasia will best be facilitated within an 'integrated' professional regulatory system.

VIII. Public health legislation

§i. *Beyond corporate exploitation of parliamentary process*

In Kafka's story *Before the Law*, a man is warned, while standing at the 'door' of the law, that beyond is a series of increasingly impenetrable barriers. In the era of the market state, such obstacles to justice could include the capacity of corporate power elites to evade application of the law, or to effectively lobby for its favourable (to them) alteration in a manner not transparent to public scrutiny. Yet the man is convinced that the system is just (or he has no practical alternative either to waiting, or to the legal system), so he waits there for years. He gives presents to the doorkeeper which are accepted 'only lest you should think you'd left some stone unturned'. Eventually, near death, the man asks the doorkeeper, 'everybody seeks the law, … so how is it that in all these years no one but me has demanded admittance?' The doorkeeper shouts at the now deaf old man, with typical Kafka-esque ambiguity: 'This entrance was meant for you alone. Now I'm going to close it.'

Like so many of Kafka's characters, this man before the impenetrable 'door' to the law has unrealistic hopes that society's institutions and rules will remain committed to foundational social virtues. Perhaps this short story paints an accurate picture of the 'window dressing' manner in which legislation supposed to protect patient rights has actually operated to defeat them in the fully privatised global health care system hypothesised here as operating in the age of the market state.

It used to be said that a major disadvantage of legislation as a form of regulation in the health care system was its relative inability to respond rapidly to complex changes in medical knowledge and circumstances. Early statutory prohibitions of human reproductive cloning, for example, failed to accurately define the actual scientific technique eventually used. Another less well explored problem with legislation as a regulatory tool in this context, however, is the ease with which corporate strategists, by means of lobbying, election campaign donations and 'revolving-door' 'staffer' appointments, can take control of a statute's aims and contents and turn them into marketing tools with an often circuitous relationship to patient benefit.

The state, under early models of its social contract pact with the medical profession, as we saw earlier, provides a subsidy for medical education and ensures a monopoly over professional service, in return for high standards of care and assistance with fulfilling its public health obligations. Legislation may be used to achieve these aims by controlling specific aspects of doctor–patient relations, or indirectly by funding public health education programs. Legislation benefits from the legal fiction of being considered the reflected will of the majority of the competent population. Legislation has a ready capacity for enforcement by the executive arm of government. It also has a good corporate 'brand' value amongst health care consumers.

In a society governed by the market state, legislation has become increasingly involved with regulating the intricacies of the doctor–patient relationship. It is also (mostly without any necessary or consistent connection) more frequently used to shape health systems so that they favour private corporate interests.

Legislation, for example, has sought to alter important aspects of the process of consent and informed consent, access to medical records and the manner and nature of diagnosis, treatment and its withdrawal. It has also, as we have seen, permitted breaches of confidentiality for socially useful purposes, such as prevention of child abuse or infectious disease or cancer, firearms offences and driving under the influence of alcohol, or public danger from epileptic attacks in those using motor vehicles. Prescription of dangerous drugs, as well as notification and certification of the birth or death of a patient, are examples of health care routinely so regulated in the public interest. Statutes, however, have also increasingly sought to control access to the doctor–patient relationship itself, the grounds of professional misconduct and the capacity of consumers to litigate against health care corporations. Religious ideology has been a factor behind certain pieces of high-profile health legislation in the era of the market state. This is possibly because public displays of commitment to such values on selected issues have been useful ways to counteract suspicions of the dominance of industry lobby groups and the profit motive in government deliberations.

Sometimes such issues have captured the public imagination (for example, stem cell research) and held the possibility of industry interests being unduly inhibited. In such circumstances, parliamentary inquiries have often been established, their representatives being selected in advance by the government on the basis that they were likely to deliver a result favourable to corporate interests. A conscience vote (not on party lines) could then be held, so that the legislature briefly represented a more genuine social contract process.

In the United States, Federal and State legislatures (in denial of the important constitutional doctrine supporting separation of legislative, judicial and executive powers) have gone as far as to rapidly draft statutes that permitted the overturning of one specific health law decision by the Florida State Supreme Court that upset religious fundamentalists. This decision had accepted a husband's legal entitlement to permit physicians to remove treatment (determined on expert clinical evidence to be 'futile') from his 39-year-old wife, who had been in a persistent vegetative state for 13 years after a cardiac arrest.[63]

In the age of the market state, proposed legislation specifying safe working hours for junior medical staff, or ensuring adequate systems of training, supervision and remuneration, has been likely to receive a lukewarm reception from the corporate sector. The chief reason isn't that private sector health care operations do not care about the welfare of their staff, their public reputation or their contribution to a safe health care system. Rather, it has been simply a matter of business priorities. To be globally competitive, private health care corporations need to either promote themselves to the limited pool of high-income consumers (as possessing cutting edge excellence worth any cost), or drive wages and conditions down and/or monopolise the market, or maintain high levels of taxpayer subsidies from the state.

As a further example, proposed statutory provisions for quality, safety and cost-effectiveness regulation that would slow biotechnology 'pipeline' development and marketing approval, or facilitate competition from generic products, have similarly been likely to be strongly lobbied against by corporate interests in private discussions with the relevant government Minister.

Beyond the age of the market state, however, health Ministers will be required to be registered as health professionals after a set period of training (necessarily more abbreviated than that of a clinician). Such training will be designed to allow them to directly experience loyalty to the relief of patient suffering in a variety of appropriate contexts with the health system. It will also require them to understand how an 'integrated' system of health professional regulation, based on virtue and fundamentally resonating with conscience, actually works in their own area of expertise. They will have trained alongside doctors, nurse-practitioners and health industry managers.

Such 'integrated' health professional training is more likely to ensure that such politicians come to legislative office with independent views about policy reform, and thus will not be so easily snowed by ministerial advisers, lobbying, lucrative promises of post-office employment, or the need to 'pay back' industry for campaign contributions.

Issues such as patient control over their own DNA samples and genetic information, care of the chronically ill, emergency care of injured citizens, access to medical services in remote areas, treatment of HIV/AIDS and response to any emerging infectious disease pandemic will provide an opportunity for a health Minister to display commitment to making health legislation coherent with both foundational principles of bioethics and international human rights. Such health legislation, having an acknowledged place in an 'integrated' professional regulatory system, will explicitly comply with the influential Limberg principles. These require that state restrictions on civil and political human rights, whilst pursuing compelling public health goals, must be incorporated in law, and be proportional and reasonably necessary to achieve that aim.[64]

At this time, public health legislation will also play an important role (as WTO rules are altered to permit a variety of global social outcomes instead of an inexorable movement to privatisation) in underpinning taxpayer-funded schemes that provide universal, citizen-funded access to basic health services, particularly in emergencies, as well as affordable essential medicines.[65] Legislation fulfilling such egalitarian policies will by this means become a global standard that forms the basis for a multilateral treaty.[66]

IX. Constitutional law: The right to health

§i. Setting basic health responsibilities for the market state

A human right to health, based on either a domestic constitution or international human rights law, will be an important means by which health professionals in the age beyond the market state may be able to calibrate (that is, evaluate for coherence with foundational professional virtues and principles) health policy and legislation.[67] The human right to health will be generally regarded as imposing duties on a market state to protect, respect and fulfil economic, social and cultural (rather than civil and political) obligations towards its citizens.

In the market state era, where health policy has generally supported full privatisation, health care corporate managers have preferred to view the international human right to health as a largely symbolic, non-individually enforceable, progressively realisable concession to normative decency, assisting a loose conglomeration of NGOs, civil society and environmental activists, so-called free trade 'flat-earthers' and 'small is beautiful' economists in their supposedly hopelessly idealistic claims to democratic legitimacy.

This denigratory 'sound-grab' mass media portrayal of any potentially influential opponents of health care privatisation has become increasingly less accurate or popular, however, as a result of cases in many jurisdictions in which a constitutional right to health has been invoked to, for example, support legal obligations on the state to provide access to affordable generic pharmaceuticals to treat HIV/AIDS,[68] or prepare for emerging infectious disease pandemics by compulsory licensing of necessary, but patented medicines, priced excessively and without accountability.

An illustrative example is the decision of the constitutional court of South Africa in *Soobramoney v Minister of Health (Kwazulu-Natal)*.[69] A 41-year-old unemployed diabetic with chronic renal failure sought regular 6 hourly use of one of the State's 20 dialysis machines. Guidelines developed by the relevant hospital limited such access to patients with acute remedial renal failure or chronic failure with good prospects for long-term quality of life. Mr Soobramoney, who was denied access, relied (unsuccessfully) on two sections of the South African Constitution 1996: section 27(3) – 'no one may be refused emergency medical treatment', and section 11 – 'everyone has the right to life'.

The court held that such rights must be interpreted with a margin of appreciation for the State's limited resources. This led to its obligations being reduced to the need to demonstrate policies attempting to progressively realise better access to health care. Nevertheless, the decision supported an important constitutional line in the sand about the limits of privatisation in health care: it should not extend, without a firm democratic mandate, into emergency or so-called catastrophic care.

The 'age of the market state' is a term that, for purposes of argument rather than as a matter of sociological fact, I have used here to refer to a period of state promotion of global privatisation that is half physically realised or imminent and half ideologically immanent in health care policy and institutions. In such conditions, health care corporations have many ways (including influencing appointments to the bench and funding protracted litigation) to ensure that any judicial interpretations of a constitutional right to health serve their financial interests (for example, by facilitating access to private health insurance). They are likely to successfully lobby that a state's obligation to progressively realise a right to health merely requires it to periodically enunciate strategies that promote effective relevant use of available health care resources, particularly 'quality' health care and 'innovative' medicines.[70] They are likely to have the ear of government when they argue that the core content of this human right, the minimum obligation that cannot be set aside, should be restricted to a state's responsibility to reduce serious threats to public health from international sources such as infectious disease pandemics or bioterrorism.

In the post-market state era, however, the international right to health is likely to be taken much more seriously in policy discussions, as an important marker of a state's obligation to fulfil its duties to provide the basic preconditions for health, such as food, water, sanitation, shelter and protection of the environment. It will also assist leaders amongst health professionals to challenge states to retain, or enhance, their responsibilities for access to health care, including emergency health care.[71]

Leaders amongst health professionals (importantly now defined to include corporate managers and policy-makers), beyond the age of the market state, are more likely to be aware that the human right to health allows only legally prescribed, non-discriminatory, proportional and least necessary restrictions on international civil and political human rights (such as freedom of movement, freedom of thought, conscience or religion, freedom of expression, freedom of peaceful assembly and freedom of association). Contentious instances will involve legislation isolating, confining or compulsorily testing potentially infected persons. Such disproportional and ineffective measures may discourage infected consumers/patients from seeking counselling and treatment or notifying others, and thus violate both civil and political human rights and the human right to health.

Such leaders will know well that a state's constitutional or international law obligations to respect the human right to physical integrity may overlap with international right to health obligations in issues such as prevention of female circumcision/genital mutilation, or risky medical research without adequate benefit to the population of subjects involved. They will likewise understand that respecting the human right to life may similarly overlap with fulfilling the human right to health in relation to reducing infant and maternal mortality and providing cost-effective access to safe, or high quality essential medicines.[72] Likewise, respect for the prohibition on inhuman and degrading treatment may be linked with fulfilling the human right to health as it affects prisoners' deprivation of medical care.[73]

Similar overlapping concerns for leaders amongst health professionals will also increasingly arise in relation to access to and safety of abortion, or the state's obligation to respect the civil and political human rights of, for example, HIV/AIDS patients, as a strategy to encourage involvement in testing, counselling, safe-sex education, partner notification and public health treatment programs. Such leaders, working within an 'integrated' system of professional regulation, will seek to demonstrate to the public that technical and financial, as well as conceptual, limitations prevent the right to health involving a justiciable guarantee to each person of a minimum level of actual health. They will ensure that legislation which has the effect of inhibiting medical research also exhibits a 'compelling interest' to interfere with the human right to health.

For present purposes, the extent to which a human right to health will be perceived by health professionals as setting standards by which consumers should be able to access basic medical care, or initiate a doctor–patient relationship, is particularly relevant. Using military force to prevent health care consumers reaching hospital, for instance, would be a clear violation of the international human right to health. So would banning women from seeing doctors, or establishing a privatised health care system that denies private insurance to women and children. A similar violation would include failing to adequately train and distribute sufficient doctors for a population's needs, or allocating a proportion of gross national product that is not sufficient to provide adequate facilities, equipment or drugs to prevent occupational and infectious disease.[74]

In the post-market state era, state reports on such matters, reviewed by the committee monitoring compliance with the international right to health in Article 12 of the *ICESCR*, will be taken much more seriously. State health policy deliberations will routinely consider this committee's assessment of, for example, the number of hospital beds, doctors and nurses relative to population and whether doctors are staying in their country of training or aggregating in urban rather than rural areas or away from low income, indigenous or other potentially marginalised groups. Institutions such as the European Court of Human Rights, relying on these reports, will play a more influential role in developing a corpus of jurisprudence concerning patient human rights related to the right to health. This body of jurisprudence will more uniformly flow into the common law through judicial decisions facilitated by legislation such as the *Human Rights Act* 1998 (UK), which requires English courts to consider the application of relevant human rights from the *ECHR* to the case before it.[75]

In the post-market state age, such factors are likely to increasingly place cultural and intellectual pressure upon judges in jurisdictions without Bills of Rights to incorporate norms such as the international right to health into domestic law, particularly where those norms have no prior constitutional specification. This incorporation may take the form of direct transformation into common law rules, use as principles to resolve legislative ambiguities, revisionist interpretations of existing constitutional guarantees, or enhanced constitutional implications.

Chapter summary and cases for further discussion

• In the age of the market state, judicial rulings and legislation have become marketing or profit-making strategies utilised by the managers of multinational corporations.

• In the era beyond the market state, the medical duty to rescue may be conceptualised as including a duty on the market state to come to the aid of vulnerable populations, for example by legislation respecting, protecting and fulfilling the preconditions for health or access to health services.

• Decision-makers using an 'integrated' approach to professional regulation are likely to try to set instances of alleged medical negligence into their structural or institutional context, rather than focusing on individual blame.

• Whether or not a doctor's failure to disclose possession of shares in – or other financial connections with – a relevant medical device or pharmaceutical or health management company is recognised by courts as having a consent-vitiating effect will be a major test of the extent to which a legal system can be relied upon to protect the interests of patients.

• In the age beyond the market state, the legal rules of informed consent will no longer be a PR exercise in 'paper compliance' involving signed and filed forms in which consumers and research subjects trade responsibilities with health care corporations.

• 'Integrated' professional regulation will favour a presumption against contract becoming the dominant form of regulation between consumer and doctor, only able to be overcome by good evidence of factors such as capacity and independent advice. Doctors will be less restricted by such contracts and associated protocols from openly discussing ethical difficulties with patients or research subjects.

• Doctors compromising patient care by accepting pharmaceutical company gifts and sponsorships may be 'caught' by fiduciary legal rules. So may a wider range of health professionals who allow third party corporations to restrict length of hospital stay, and/or deny marginal or expensive treatments, investigations or referrals.

- In the age beyond the market state, an 'integrated' system of regulating medical professionalism will be more able to ensure that its principles and rules support a 'space' where patient trust and physician loyalty to the relief of suffering can flourish under the protection and respect of the state. Particularly relevant in this context will be the legal doctrines of confidentiality and privilege of doctor–patient communications.

- Creation of a constitutional right to taxpayer-funded emergency treatment, as well as a multilateral treaty on universal health care and health technology evaluation, will become important means of welcoming multinational health care corporations into negotiations for a revitalised global social contract supporting foundational professional virtues and principles.

Case study: Joan's story

An intern saw a 65-year-old lady, Joan, with a history of jejunal bypass for obesity and subsequent constant diarrhoea, which she treated symptomatically. Though she'd lost weight, she was still 140kg when she presented with a lesion of her caecum/ascending colon. This was thought to be colon cancer. 'She doesn't do a thing,' said one family member. 'She's an alcoholic and she can't cut down,' said another. 'That's consumed all her life, that anger.' 'She's got no tolerance for other people.' 'She's actually asked me to book the funeral.' 'If you sent her to rehab, not that she can afford it, she'd just walk out after punching everybody.' Joan consented to a right hemicolectomy and repair of an incisional hernia from her jejunal bypass surgery. She was very difficult to intubate and central venous access was obtained only after her subclavian artery had been punctured. After two hours of general anaesthesia the operation commenced. The surgeon noted massive adhesions and repaired the right hemicolectomy. While checking the liver and spleen for metastases, he noted large stones in the gall bladder. The patient had not consented to a cholecystectomy, but owing to the risk of more adhesions and her high anaesthetic risk, her gall bladder was removed. Despite a positive outcome for the patient, the surgeon was later hauled before the hospital's clinical practice manager and threatened with being 'kicked off the plan' if he ever 'exposed' his institution like that again. If the effective workplace enforcer of standards of medical professionalism is a corporate official, how will this influence the professional values of junior doctors? How could such clinical decision-making be better regulated?

Case study: Glenda's story

An 80-year-old woman called Glenda had been rescheduled to have a day-stay aortic-bifemoral angiogram, plus percutaneous transluminal angioplasty of her right leg. She suffered an acute intra-abdominal bleed requiring admission to the ICU. Glenda lived in a privatised aged care facility and had a history of cerebrovascular accidents, bowel resection and stoma formation, atrial fibrillation and longstanding peripheral vascular disease. 'The poor old thing,' said a senior clinician to his junior house staff, 'is moderately deaf, has mild cognitive impairment and has no one to visit her. Doctors, as you know, don't like to visit nursing homes much these days. Anyway, Glenda says she is worried about the risks of untreated pain and more bleeding when she returns to the nursing home. "I am old," she tells me. "I don't need to walk far, so why bother?" Keeping her here is eating into her life savings. Should we ask her relatives or some corporate philanthropist for sufficient money to keep her alive? The Emergency Department has recently received a patient with major trauma who needs but is unable to secure an ICU bed.' What issues are raised here for medical professional regulation and how should they best be resolved?

MEDICAL
PROFESSIONALISM
IN
THE
MODERN
ARMED
CONFLICT
ZONE

I. Medical professionalism, torture and corporate-controlled wars

§i. Torture's direct conflict with medical professionalism

In Orwell's *1984*, a man is taken (without being formally arrested or tried) by the Thought Police to be tortured in the Ministry of Love. He is indoctrinated to believe there is no loyalty except loyalty to the Party. He is forced to reveal and debase the most critical interests in his life narrative. His conscience nevertheless resonates with one intuitive conviction: that there is some 'principle' in the universe that will supplant the cruelty of his oppressors. To overcome this last emotive barrier to obedience, the man is exposed to his greatest fear. He pleads, as is intended, for that torture to be done to someone else – the person he loves most.

This section considers how an 'integrated' system of professional regulation should respond to use by the market state of torture and warfare. For this purpose, modern instances such as physician involvement in torture at Abu Ghraib prison in Iraq or Guantanamo Bay may be more instructive than historical examples of doctors at Soviet psychiatric institutions interning healthy persons involuntarily for political purposes, or South African physicians acquiescing in the death in custody of anti-apartheid activists.

Many international human rights norms creating a duty on the market state to 'respect' individuals, including patients, can be derogated from on grounds of the overriding need to protect public health. This is not the case with the international civil and political human right requiring a state to 'refrain' from torture, or cruel, unusual or degrading treatment or punishment.[1] Article 1 of the *Torture Convention* defines torture as state infliction of pain and suffering for political purposes. Common examples include sham executions, sexual assault, prolonged arbitrary detention with sleep and sensory deprivation, application of electric shocks, water immersion, disfigurement, infliction of pain and humiliation, disappearance, or threats against a loved one and forced witnessing of others' torture.

The prohibition on torture is a peremptory norm of international law with the character of *jus cogens*. Within an 'integrated' regulatory system, *jus cogens* norms could be viewed as the few principles that have been supported unreservedly by all nations (prohibitions on slavery and genocide are two others) in a type of official recognition of the Kantian categorical imperative for particular situations.[2] Violation of such a principle fundamentally contradicts the basic social and professional virtues which underpin international civil society and is prohibited by laws which attract jurisdiction by the courts of any state.[3] This is true regardless of the supposed community benefit (for example in the so-called War on Terror) allegedly derived from the torture. Policies or legislation supporting institutionalised torture, or cruel treatment, also presumptively violate the market state's duty to 'fulfil' its citizens' human right to health. The prohibition on torture extends to a state's duty to 'protect' patients against torture performed by 'private' persons.[4] This definition includes private corporations who run gaols and detention centres, charging the state for provision of such a service.

Beyond the age of the market state the community will rely on leaders of medical professionalism to be open in their critical analysis of the advantages the state claims from sophisticated redefinitions of torture and from 'outsourcing' its practice to private contractors. A major issue here may be the state's refusal to accept direct responsibility, due to the problematic place that corporations and their employees have under international and domestic human rights law.

Health professionals, broadly conceived, will fail to honour the fundamental principles of medical professionalism if they – or the health system they support – neglect to investigate torture (according, for example, to the *Istanbul Protocol*), particularly amongst patients at high risk, such as refugees (sometimes referred to as 'illegal immigrants' by market states).[5] They will also do so if they do not take patient allegations of torture seriously, if they inhibit patient disclosure of torture by exhibiting discomfort, and if they remain unduly reticent about promoting related human rights.

In 1982, a UN Declaration set out principles of medical ethics prohibiting physician involvement in, or certification of prisoners as fit for, torture or other cruel, inhuman or degrading treatment or punishment.[6] The use of physicians in torture is particularly obnoxious because their presence, according to traditional canons of professionalism, implies to patients a concern with the relief of, rather than an infliction of, suffering. The market state's imminent capacity for ubiquitous and highly efficient nanotechnology surveillance and data storage makes protection of such basic human rights an even more important task for the leaders of medical professionalism.

§ii. Medical leadership against cruel and degrading treatment and punishment

Victor Frankl's *Man's Search for Meaning* describes a physician's experience in Nazi concentration camps during World War II. This doctor, like those at the Abu Ghraib or Guantanamo Bay prisons, witnessed the systematic blunting of inmates' emotions, intrinsic dignity, conscience and humanity through subjection to starvation, exposure and exhaustion, as well as random and incessant cruelty and suffering. Prisoners were thus desensitised to the constant fear of death, to longing for home and family, to disgust itself. They could, however, still be roused to indignation at the injustice of being beaten or insulted by guards for being lazy, or lacking in the spirit of comradeship.

Human rights obliging the state to prohibit cruel, unusual and degrading treatment and punishment are conceptually distinct from those dealing with torture under international law. They have not yet, however, been generally recognised as constituting a peremptory norm of *jus cogens*. Neither are they the subject of a separate international convention. Yet they provide a very important protection for patients, particularly by shaping the outer limits of acceptable medical practice in a health system dominated by market state interests.

In *Case of D v United Kingdom*, for example, the European Court of Human Rights held that deportation of an HIV/AIDS infected patient to his country of origin (a developing country) was state conduct which violated his human right to be protected from inhuman or degrading treatment or punishment. The judges reasoned that such deportation would result in his being denied adequate medical treatment and exposed to poor public health conditions.[7] Laws requiring involuntary testing, isolation, segregation and surveillance of patients infected with a highly contagious disease could also be calibrated by health professionals as presumptively violating the human right requiring the state to protect patients from cruel, unusual or degrading treatment or punishment.

Leaders of medical professionalism may likewise be able to use such international human rights protections to oppose certain cost-cutting denials of treatment. They would also be relevant to a health professional's coherence reasoning concerning legislation that reintroduces or continues capital punishment.

Physician participation in capital punishment, particularly through methods involving medical skill and technology (such as lethal injection), is fundamentally opposed to the primary professional virtue of loyalty to the relief of patient suffering. The profession has a long tradition of opposition to such involvement, which extends to legal proceedings and protests against the state and its institutions.[8] The Guatemalan Doctors' and Surgeons' Association (*Colegio de Médicos y Cirujanos de Guatemala*), as but one example, in an act of particularly courageous civil disobedience, issued a public notice announcing its refusal to obey a law requiring execution by lethal injection, based on the duty to preserve life enunciated in the *Hippocratic Oath*.[9]

It could be argued that lethal injection is coherent with principles of medical professionalism, on the basis that it is amongst the methods of execution that cause less suffering. On many occasions, however, finding a vein is difficult, intravenous lines clog, and the death process can last up to half an hour or more. Patients may choke, gasp, heave and show other signs of pain and discomfort. At the execution of Tommie Black in 1996 in Indiana, for example, physicians were forced to insert a central line (that is, a cannula into a large vein, such as the internal jugular, subclavian or femoral), which took over 35 minutes, while the patient remained conscious.

If a doctor is called to a botched or 'flawed' execution where the patient remains alive only by mischance, adherence to medical professionalism foundational virtues and principles demands that a physician begin full resuscitation. An exception may arise where the patient has prepared a non-coerced advance directive against that course. If the criminal justice system is anything but scrupulously fair and impartial, the death penalty may be perceived as violating the human right of freedom from arbitrary deprivation of life and, of course, the right to respect for human dignity. The death penalty is particularly problematic in terms of coherence with foundational social and professional virtues when it is imposed by a market state. With what authority, for example, could a government widely understood to be preferentially at the service of corporate interests rather than citizens, be able to take the life of people it terms 'consumers'?

A related area of potential conflict for the doctor loyal to the relief of patient suffering is the political prisoner hunger strike. The patient is here engaged in an act of civil disobedience or protest. The medical professional involved will have to balance respect for patient autonomy with bioethical and international human rights principles against cruel treatment or punishment. Legislation which requires medical treatment (including force feeding) in this situation, without free consent, may also contravene the international human rights requirement of Article 7 of the *ICCPR*. Leaders of medical professionalism may seek guidance in resolving such issues from the publications of UN committees monitoring relevant human rights norms.

11. Biosecurity and militarisation of the market state

§1. *Problems in corrupt or failed states*

In market states that have become corrupt, rather than wicked (actively promoting evil), officials may find it useful to appear to support generally accepted moral and ethical principles, and even international human rights, in public. Such actions will be good for staff morale and investor confidence. Yet, in relative secrecy, such officers are likely to disregard any obligations and responsibilities, in the creation and application of policy, that would interfere with their personal and corporate special interests. This approach may be implicitly promoted in developing nations that are required, by IMF and World Bank free market fundamentalist policies, to open up domestic markets to foreign capital, or are given large amounts of foreign aid or postwar reconstruction funds in advance of established governance systems.

In a developing society where politicians, the police, judges, the military, patent officers, health technology regulators and scientific researchers are open to bribery by multinational corporations, health care privatisation may proceed smoothly, though with substantial risks to the health of local and international communities. The rulers of such corrupt states may see personal advantage in indirectly or directly promoting, for example, regional political instability and even bioterrorism.

Amidst such institutionalised corruption, it could be argued, professionals showing leadership by consistently implementing core principles of medical professionalism in the face of obstacles risk being denigrated by state officials, having privileges, staff and facilities withdrawn, or even being murdered or 'disappeared'. A corrupt state, in a worst-case scenario, may also enforce such policies by election fraud, and by manipulating the judiciary – through case assignment, and bribing officials to give particular verdicts, lose files, and delay, or drop, cases.

In such circumstances, health professionals (as an influential knowledge elite) may be encouraged to display obsequious quietism, or deference to corporate corruption of the judiciary, legislature, security officers or bureaucracy. Those with qualms and disturbances of conscience, who resist and/or speak out against this process and the suffering it causes, will be asked to remain loyal and not withdraw or exit from the system. Any who do decide to resign or depart in protest are likely to be pressured to announce that this is for largely concocted 'family' or 'personal' reasons, and to not make public their 'insider' knowledge of fraud and abuse of power.

War and terrorism create additional stresses on health professionals in such corrupt societies who attempt to encourage the state to fulfil its basic responsibilities under humanitarian and international human rights law. The remarkable thing is that so many health professionals remain, and are likely to continue to remain, willing to rise to these challenges, even at the cost of their own lives. Medical professionalism is often practised with greater commitment to fundamental virtues and principles in failed states or nations with serious civil unrest than in more outwardly stable developed states.

It could be objected that a professional regulatory system which predicates not only obedience to, but the legitimate existence of, legal rules on critical reflection about conscience or foundational social or professional virtues encourages a seemingly anarchic or iconoclastic approach to governance that could itself facilitate social anarchy, failed states and threats from disaffected scientists doing 'dual use' research. Any legislature's members, in a corrupt state, will be naturally prejudiced against professionals attempting to manufacture an artificial regulatory coherence between vague internationalist ideals and existing laws that such politicians claim an electoral mandate to pass. Scientists motivated by vengeful religious ideologies to spread contagion are unlikely to be effectively restrained solely through education about codes of conduct.

Such arguments might also allege that an 'integrated' professional regulatory system, with its emphasis on foundational ideals, is merely an exercise in cultural imperialism, distanced from the varying realities of a particular nation's social and historical context. Health professionals are a wealthy elite who have often been influenced by their education abroad away from an understanding of the religious, cultural and security imperatives that must influence government policy in the real world.

Yet the transfer of allegiance from the corrupt market states, with their systematic and accelerated dismantling of social capital and citizen involvement in policy, to cosmopolitan groupings based around shared values (not restricted by geographical or cultural boundaries) could be one of the positive governance outcomes of the era of corporate sovereignty. For this to occur, some socially influential groups must constantly raise the public profile of such ideals. The argument being made here is that health professionals are well positioned to assume that important role.

§ii. *Genocide, slavery, the arms trade and forensic investigations*

In Albert Camus' *The Plague*, the fictional Dr Rieux tends suffering patients in the 'absurd' situation of a town closed by law because of plague. He is living in a 'fortress world', one possible scenario for a fully privatised global health care system, in which the increasing divide between rich and poor is solved by military-enforced separation. Dr Rieux struggles to accept the fact that his chief professional task now seems less to relieve suffering than to enforce state quarantine legislation with the help of soldiers. He wrestles with what sustains him. Perhaps, he muses, it is 'common decency', 'doing my job', 'being a man', or the 'path of sympathy'.

One of the unfortunate social consequences of monetarist and/or free market fundamentalist ideologies is that economic stability is dependent on large amounts of public (taxpayer) money being spent by the market state on the production of military weapons, many carefully designed to destroy all human life. Others (such as 'butterfly' landmines) are constructed to maim children and terrify populations.

Given the growing unemployment, poverty and illness promoted by their free market fundamentalist policies, market states also may need to spend increasing amounts on both mass media propaganda and on arms and military expenditure, in order to maintain power over an increasingly dissatisfied populace. Such expenditure will be promoted by the corporations receiving it as having the added bonus of stabilising economic growth. It is important that the basic canons of medical professionalism sanction the capacity of health professionals to continue to challenge such policies in the interests of public health.

In this context, physicians will have increasingly important tasks in terms of documenting human rights violations, through forensic investigation and expert testimony. The physical dangers and problems of mixed loyalties for physicians performing such roles are significant. Whether they involve attempting to identify and establish cause of death at mass grave exhumations, uncovering the source of a bioterrorist disease outbreak, investigating deaths in police custody, or documenting ill-treatment and torture of detainees, doctors in such circumstances must be aware that though a state's legal system may require their impartiality, the tenets of medical professionalism demand an informed and active professional conscience.

In El Salvador, Chile, Uruguay, the Philippines, Israel, Guatemala, Rwanda and the former Yugoslavia, for example, Physicians for Human Rights collected evidence of, and assisted those suffering after, executions, torture, mass rape and attempted genocide. Its representatives gathered forensic evidence concerning the massacre by Serbian troops of Croatian patients and medical staff at the Vukovar hospital. In Cambodia, Mozambique and Somalia, health professionals with this NGO assembled data on the effects of landmines on a civilian population. They helped track down abducted and displaced persons through genetic family tracing in El Salvador.

Testifying in a court of law is a well-accepted duty of medical professionalism. Medical testimony establishing the identity of victims of torture, 'ethnic cleansing', terrorism or military atrocities often has to use genetic evidence. Though DNA 'genetic fingerprinting' may no longer be regarded as the ultimate forensic identifier, it will undoubtedly be of increasing importance to criminal law enforcement in and beyond the era of the market state. Its role is likely to be enhanced by ubiquitous nanotechnology surveillance systems, expansion of DNA forensic databases, possibly to include either all citizens or those alleged or proven to have committed even relatively minor crimes, as well as techniques such as 'genetic profiling', which attempt to fit criminal characteristics to particular genomes.

Revelations of conflict of interest in such areas will be particularly discomforting, then, for leaders of medical professionalism. One high-profile example concerned proof that Sir Richard Doll, the eminent epidemiologist (who established statistically that smoking causes lung cancer), had been receiving consultancy fees in the 1980s from the Monsanto corporation. Monsanto was then a major chemical company, but is now involved in globally converting farmers into corporate rent payers through aggressive marketing and patent protection of its non-renewable genetically modified (GM) crops. While so employed, Sir Richard gave expert testimony to an Australian Royal Commission (without disclosing any conflict of interest) that there was no evidence that cancer had been caused by the US military's use of the defoliant Agent Orange (made by Monsanto) in the Vietnam War.[10] This evidence, now known to be false, was instrumental in restricting the compensation paid to victims (military and civilian) of this biological warfare.

III. Medical leadership and violations of patient human rights

§i. Supporting human rights and civil liberties, even under threat

In Ingmar Bergman's film *The Seventh Seal*, a medieval knight encounters a young girl, iron chains chafing her neck and arms, being taken by cart for burning at the stake in the pine forest. Her alleged crimes are intercourse with the devil and causing the plague. The knight is warned by a seedy monk against talking to this 'witch'. Instead, he touches her gently and asks about the identity of the 'evil one', understanding that she is deluded, exhausted and probably the victim of recent rape or seduction. He offers a potion to stop her pain, and water from his palm. The knight questions the soldiers about who crushed her hands and demands that the monk explain the disappearance of the girl's baby. The knight and his squire feel their consciences rage at the cruelty of this faux justice. Personified Death asks the knight, 'Don't you ever stop asking questions?'

For present purposes, we may imagine the knight to be a representative of Physicians for Human Rights or Médecins Sans Frontières, International Physicians for the Prevention of Nuclear War or the Medical Society for Prevention of War. He replies, 'No, I'll never stop.'

Interpreting this knight to be a doctor and the girl the contemporary equivalent of a witch (perhaps someone jailed and tortured as a terrorist, without a prompt and fair trial), how should we characterise, in terms of medical professionalism, the activation of conscience which so powerfully motivated him to intervene? The girl's suffering was caused not by traditional precipitants of doctor–patient relations such as infection, accidental trauma or some abnormality of physiology or anatomy. Instead, it arose from a failure by the state to consistently respect, fulfil or protect something intrinsically meaningful in the humanity of the individual. Just what this something is has become the subject of the developing corpus of international human rights – increasingly revered by the oppressed and marginalised people of the world, but not necessarily by medical professionals, health policy-makers, or officials of the market state.

As well as prohibitions of torture, or cruel, inhuman or degrading treatment or punishment, civil and political international human rights relevant to medical professionalism, as previously discussed, require the protection of human dignity and equality, of the human right to life, of free consent to medical and scientific treatment, of physical integrity, of non-discrimination, of freedom to receive and impart information, and of freedom from arbitrary interference with privacy. Application of many of these norms to issues concerning, for example, abortion, euthanasia or privacy of information is likely to benefit from judicial interpretation of similar constitution-based human rights.

To what extent should medical professionalism and leadership encourage doctors and health policy workers to become human rights promoters and advocates for individual patients, either those they already have a professional relationship with, or those for whom their conscience has been specifically awakened?[11] What is the wider professional duty of a doctor who suspects a patient's/consumer's suffering is caused by, for example, child, spouse or elder abuse, the state's systematic use of violence, torture, rape, displacement, disappearance and genocide against a civilian population, or racial and sexual discrimination?

The United Nations has enunciated norms of medical professionalism that prohibit physician involvement in, or certification of prisoners as fit for, torture or other cruel, inhuman or degrading treatment or punishment.[12] Similarly important international human rights norms require that medical practitioners assist in preventing the global problems of child abuse and trafficking, the market state's systematic use of violence, torture, rape, displacement, disappearance and genocide against a civilian population, and racial and sexual discrimination.

As we move beyond the era of the market state, it will be even less acceptable for health professionals to refer to one of the million or so women and girls under 18 trafficked yearly for prostitution as a health care 'consumer'. Likewise, it will be unsuitable to consider any of the world's 10 million refugees, or 5 million internally displaced persons, as willing participants in the ideology of free market fundamentalism. Can the term 'health care consumer' really be said to apply to victims of any one the 35 or so wars currently raging across the earth, or of state-promoted torture or rape in the guise of 'ethnic cleansing', or to any of the 250 million children exploited for labour, sexual gratification or as soldiers, or the 1.2 billion people living in severe poverty, without adequate obstetric care, food, safe water or sanitation? If the term 'health care consumer' is not capable of application to such a wide range of persons in need of access to health care, why should it be acceptable at all as an important descriptor in health policy decisions?

This conclusion is even more true if we realise that gender discrimination, poverty, famine and displacement by warfare are significant factors in large numbers of children in African countries still failing to receive basic information from health professionals about how to avoid infection with HIV/AIDS, despite often over 30 per cent of the population being seropositive.

Health professionals, with their social status, education and political influence, are well positioned to become human rights promoters and advocates in relation to this type of patient suffering. Health policy-makers may also become promoters of economic, social and cultural human rights in regard to a whole population, in connection with, for example, issues such as prevention of nuclear war, the use of biological or chemical weapons, reduction in third world debt or facilitation of the production or import of cheap generic pharmaceuticals.[13] Such political activity of behalf of the global community of patients is likely to become a more dominant focus for leaders of medical professionalism in the post-market state age.[14]

A major problem with using international law to protect the civil, political, economic, social and cultural human rights of patients/consumers in a fully privatised global health care system is that such norms are chiefly addressed to states. States are traditionally not responsible for protecting citizens from private violations by other individuals ('individual', in this sense, is a legal concept that includes corporate entities). Increased efforts have been made, however, to hold states accountable where their legal rules and political policies have acquiesced in, or not shown due diligence in preventing, third party (for example, corporate) actions which, if performed by the state, would constitute human rights violations. The human right to life has been held to include a state duty to protect an individual from the criminal acts of another.[15]

Human rights advocacy by health professionals is encouraged by, amongst others, the *Journal of the American Medical Association* (*JAMA*) which, since 1983, has dedicated the first issue every August to such topics. UN instruments such as the *Declaration* and proposed *Convention on the Rights of Disabled Persons*, as well as instruments such as those relating to the abolition of the death penalty, rely heavily on physicians for effective implementation. New responsibilities may include helping patients who have exhausted domestic legal remedies to formally and directly complain to international human rights committees under optional protocols to international human rights conventions.[16]

§ii. *Medical professionalism and international humanitarian law*

In his book *The Last and First Men*, Olaf Stapledon describes how various generations of human beings destroy the civilisations they have created through an inability to progress their moral and spiritual development in parallel with their technological accomplishments. A related theme of *Who Owns Our Health?* is to support the natural law position that conscience and striving for virtue are an inescapable better part of human nature, even in the most extreme circumstances. The argument has been made that no regulatory system seeking community legitimacy can afford not to champion justice, human dignity and loyalty to the relief of patient suffering. Indeed, herein lies much of the ongoing global support for international humanitarian law.

The conceptual foundations of medical professionalism have a strong historical connection with international humanitarian law.[17] The *Geneva Conventions* in 1949, the *Hague Convention* of 1907, the *Genocide Convention* and the *Nuremberg Charter* all impose upon states positive duties to permit, and negative duties to not hinder, the exercise of medical professionalism amidst armed conflict. These have now achieved status as customary international law.[18]

Three illustrative foundational principles created by such humanitarian law instruments are neutrality in prioritisation of treatment, treatment only for patients' benefit, and treatment in accordance with generally accepted medical standards. The latter do not refer to whatever (possibly abysmal) professional standards may exist in a particular state, or be endorsed by it as justified by an alleged exigency such as a war on terror. They refer instead to the ethical principles set out in codes such as the modern restatement of the *Hippocratic Oath* and the *International Code of Medical Ethics*.[19]

NGOs such as the International Red Cross, Physicians for Human Rights[20] and Médecins Sans Frontières,[21] though often focused on relief of individual patient suffering in the context of armed conflict, are increasingly involved in monitoring, preventing, alleviating and even defining state violations of international humanitarian law.

The guiding ethical principles of both the International Red Cross and Médecins Sans Frontières indicate their strong commitment to professional conscience. In the latter instance they are first, *le devoir d'ingérence* or the duty to interfere regardless of any principle of state sovereignty, second, 'real, direct, immediate and fervid' medical action (*action vécue*), third, publicity of the violation and of such action, and fourth, 'efficiency of the medical act' so that it does not endanger the organisation's own staff.[22] Many in such NGOs, along with non-physician groups such as Amnesty International and Human Rights Watch, see themselves as at the vanguard of a cosmopolitan world order governed by both international humanitarian law and the *Universal Declaration of Human Rights*.

The non-government organs of humanitarian law have deep concerns about bioweapons and chemical weapons research proceeding in secret, without the possibility of beneficial 'spin-off' technology transfer to developing nations. Such research itself presents a grave threat to world peace and security and related treaty and humanitarian law prohibitions, and should be part of any global social contract negotiation concerning medical professionalism.

Chapter summary and cases for further discussion

- Use of torture fundamentally contradicts the basic social and professional virtues which underpin international civil society, and is prohibited by laws which attract jurisdiction by the courts of any state. This is true regardless of the supposed community benefit (in the so-called War on Terror, for example) allegedly derived from the torture.

- Laws requiring involuntary testing, isolation, segregation and surveillance of patients infected with a highly contagious emergent infectious disease appear to violate the human right requiring state restraint from cruel, unusual or degrading treatment.

- Health professionals and policy-makers have a responsibility to humanity to challenge a state's capacity to use faux judicial proceedings to impose the death penalty on those it disapproves of.

- In a developing society where politicians, police, judges, the military, patent officers, health technology regulators and scientific researchers are open to bribery by multinational corporations, health care privatisation may proceed smoothly, but with substantial risks to the health of local and international communities.

- Scientists motivated by vengeful religions ideologies to spread contagion through manipulation of 'dual use' research are unlikely to be effectively restrained solely through education about codes of conduct.

- Given the growing unemployment, poverty and illness promoted by their free market fundamentalist policies, market states may need to spend increasing amounts on both mass media propaganda and on arms and military expenditure, in order to maintain power over an increasingly dissatisfied populace.

- Health professionals, with their social status, education and political influence, are well positioned to become human rights promoters and advocates, as well as agents implementing international humanitarian law.

Case study: Salaam's story

A medical student on the way to his final exam in Burma saw a person shot by security forces in the street. He painted a red cross on his clothing and jumped off the bus to attempt cardiopulmonary resuscitation, but was himself shot dead. Any reporting of the event, locally and internationally, was prevented. What should be the content and source of the principles guiding the responsibilities of local and international medical professionals and health policy-makers in this case?

Case study: Asad's story

Asad was a medical researcher in a country subject to military coup instigated by various corporate interests opposed to the reforms of a democratically elected leader. Asad fled to neighbouring nation with his family. He knew he was leaving behind many patients who were unlikely to get adequate care, but felt his connections with the previous regime would make him a target for assassination. Should Asad's action be criticised as contrary to basic principles of medical professionalism? Should Asad be investigated by security services in his new country as a posing a risk of bioterrorism, and if so, according to what principles?

7

MANAGED
CARE
AND
THE
GLOBAL
PUBLIC–PRIVATE
DEBATE

I. Liberalising global health care

§i. *Managed or universal health care?*

'Imagine,' said an elderly woman whose family had just sold her house to finance a place in a private nursing home, 'that someone, a stranger, calls on you and says that tomorrow, or maybe in a fortnight, you'll be taken, for your own good, to a place you've never seen, to live the rest of your life. You'd end up sitting there, and thinking, after a while, just as I did, "So it has happened. I'm in a home, I'm old, feeble and this system has taken all the financial resources my husband and I spent our lives acquiring. I could never have imagined it."'[1]

This chapter seeks to apply an 'integrated' system of medical professional regulation to very specific problems associated with the global privatisation of health care. By exploring the origins and structural features of some of those issues, it seeks to map how leaders amongst health professionals may assist in shifting health systems' practice, governance and policy beyond the asymmetries of political power – and the imbalances in bureaucratic and technical knowledge

– that promoted patient vulnerability in the age of the market state.

Commitment by individual leaders amongst health professionals to virtues such as justice and loyalty to the relief of patient suffering has in the past led to valuable health policy initiatives whose time may come again. One important example occurred in the United States with the establishment of the community-based Western Clinic in Tacoma, Washington in 1910.[2] Similarly significant was Dr Michael Shadid's organisation of a cooperative health plan in Elk City, Oklahoma in 1929. Farmers purchased shares of $50 to raise capital for a new hospital, in return for receiving medical care at a discount.[3]

Such community health care initiatives were generally opposed by the American Medical Association and many State medical societies, chiefly on the basis that their apparent socialism and guild mentality were detrimental to the professional monopolies and incomes of members. Dr Shadid consequently lost his membership in the county medical society and was threatened with having his licence to practise suspended.

The transformation of the reformist impulse behind such schemes into that leading to the US profit-driven system of corporatised medicine, or managed care, was an important policy phenomenon in the late 20th century, and it provided much of the blueprint for a globalised model of private, profit-driven health care. Managed care, in general terms, involves doctors employed by mostly for-profit HMOs, providing professional services to pools of consumers who are presumed to prefer private health insurance and the choice involved with low tax rates to contributing higher taxation to government-controlled universalist systems that provide quality health care equally to all.

In the age of the market state, corporations have found it convenient to attribute the capacity of doctors to relieve patient suffering as in large part due to the innovation and efficiency of HMOs and new health technology. The preferred business model for global privatisation of health care has involved a few corporate multinationals that as well as funding the relevant basic medical research, also aggressively patent the resultant knowledge, market and distribute it and then organise its consumption through contractual employment controls over panels of physician providers operating in hospitals owned and managed by those same companies.

Such corporations have promoted themselves, through public relations consultants, as good global citizens. Glossy brochures advertise their various philanthropic programs, corporate responsibility initiatives and ethical ratings. Staff are encouraged to believe that their work is for the benefit of humanity. But any legislated requirement that such efforts be systematically tracked, compared against competitors and publicised, has been vigorously resisted. Employees have tended to be ostracised or dismissed if they point out the inconsistency between such altruistic corporate programs and the company's dominant focus on attracting investment capital and reducing costs.

The CEOs of such multinational corporations have no doubt been aware of the social dislocation and individual harm likely to be created by a substantially privatised health care system, but have probably been comforted by the belief that this is a transitory market adjustment. Further, it has been, unfortunately, a violation of their fiduciary obligations to shareholders to prioritise social justice, for instance, or respect for human dignity, ahead of profitability. In fact, their corporate performance indicators have made it more rational for them to spend billions of dollars on marketing and advertising – 'branding' – their products and creating consumer desire for them than on improving quality of service for all citizens. Such priorities have also led to collusion and use of various business strategies to obtain monopoly prices, while minimising taxation obligations.

In the age of the market state, governments have tried to reduce budget deficits by excluding increasing numbers of citizens from taxpayer-funded 'safety net' access to health care programs. Even for middle income households, 'consumer choice' employer-provided health insurance plans have become increasingly expensive. Despite economic growth (on traditional narrow measures such as GDP), there has been little or no increase in real wages or salaries, a substantial cause being the rising cost of health care. In fact, it seems that although countries with substantially privatised health care systems have spent a greater proportion of GDP on health, their population health outcomes have been worse than those of nations running universalist (or taxpayer-funded) health care schemes.

Increasingly, the income of health care corporate executives seems disproportionate to shareholder returns, and to their contribution to health technology innovation and improved population health care outcomes. In 2006, for example, Hank McKinnell was forced to resign as CEO of the Pfizer pharmaceutical company. Pfizer was then 31st on the FORTUNE 500 list and the world's largest drug company, with yearly sales of US$51 billion (this is more than the GDP of 123 nations). Yet its bestselling product, the cholesterol-lowering drug Lipitor (technical name atorvastatin), generating annual revenue of US$12.9 billion, had not been researched and developed by Pfizer's own scientists, but merely acquired in a 2000 bidding war to purchase Warner-Lambert for $84 billion.

In fact, McKinnell, who has a PhD in business from Stanford University in California, had transformed Pfizer into a massive global financial holding company with a portfolio of 'blockbuster' (high sales volume) drugs. Unfortunately, some of the most important of these 'blockbusters' had core product patents which were soon to expire, and major safety concerns (for instance Viagra, Zoloft and Celebrex).

During McKinnell's term as CEO, Pfizer shares declined to $25.97 from their original $46, meaning that the company lost $137 billion in market value. Nevertheless, on retirement, he received $200 million.[4] This included a life pension of about $6.65 million a year, $78 million in deferred compensation, $18.3 million in performance-based shares, $12 million in severance pay, $5.8 million of vested stock grants, a $2.15 million bonus, $576,573 worth of medical, dental and life insurance and continued medical and dental coverage under Pfizer's retiree plans, as well as the cost of financial counselling programs and $305,644 for unused vacation days.

Beyond the age of the market state, health insurance companies will no longer be major drivers of global health policy. Their activities will be encouraged as valuable adjuncts to universal health care schemes, but they will be carefully regulated to ensure that they do not inequitably seek to minimise their expenses by screening out applicants who are at high risk of expensive treatment, or by charging them higher premiums, imposing co-payments or deductibles, or by asking for uncapped taxpayer subsidies. Once most health care systems in the world become privatised, citizens and health policy-makers will increasingly realise that they can no longer blame inefficiencies on the alleged shortcomings of government control, or citizen funding, of health care. Even after the most zealous attempts to create ideologically perfect free market conditions, the gap between public demand for expensive, best practice medical interventions and the capacity of health professionals and policy-makers to deliver them will continue to increase.

Medical practitioners now working in privatised hospitals will continue to be required by contracts, even more than they were in public-funded facilities, to implement rationing directly at the clinical 'coal face' – through hospital departmental budgets, staffing cuts, reductions in leave and research entitlements, audits of drug and equipment purchasing, as well as protocols controlling work practices. Health policy-makers and citizens will generally begin to suspect that this global form of managed health care is more about managing costs and liabilities than about delivering a quality service to the community.

In such a context, coherence reasoning about the foundational principles of medical professionalism should prompt doctors in positions of responsibility (for example Directors of Emergency Departments or Intensive Care Units) to let state officials, the general community and relevant hospital administrators know the limits of resource rationing below which a professional standard of care cannot be achieved. A social contract debate about global health care rationing may reinvigorate community interest in government retaining strong policy levers over the cost of health care delivery (such as reference pricing over 'innovative' health technologies and procedures).

One policy alternative may be to allow communities to vote to adopt either one standardised universalist or one privatised health care model. Another option involves rationing by listing fundable health care priorities created after community discussion (the 'Oregon experiment').[5] A revitalised commitment to medical professionalism also may see leaders amongst health professionals (including corporate executives and policy-makers) actively support arrangements whereby they periodically restrict their remuneration in accordance with patient capacity to pay, or do honorary (*pro bono*) work (in their respective fields), coming face-to-face with individual human suffering in needy communities. This may be one positive outcome of their regulatory system's emphasis on conscience, which will flow through into improved lifestyle and work value choices for the majority of health professionals.

§ii. Undoing the World Trade Organization's (WTO's) privatisation agenda on global health care

In Solzhenitsyn's *One Day in the Life of Ivan Denisovich*, early one morning a prisoner in one of Stalin's Siberian concentration camps visits the clean, white dispensary. The medical assistant is making a fair copy of a new long poem. He looks up and says that he can only exempt two men from work and their names are already written down under the greenish glass on his desk. The assistant has no medical training. He offers the prisoner a choice: if you stay and the doctor finds you ill, you'll be exempted from work duty. If you are found fit, you'll be locked up. The prisoner says nothing, but pulls his hat over his eyes and walks out. 'How can you expect,' he thinks, 'a man who's warm to understand a man who's cold?'

In the decades following World War II, many hoped that the regime of international human rights would become an important means of encouraging states to make respect for the inherent dignity of all being humans an achievable political ideal. The widespread hope was that such a commitment would mark the start of a new global social contract. It would lead to government policies that gradually reduced warfare, poverty, corruption, environmental degradation and infringements of civil and political liberties. UN human rights institutions and NGOs were to play crucial roles in this process. So too was the capacity for individual citizens to petition human rights committees and courts concerning violations of patient human rights.

Yet somehow, since that time the WTO has been able to create a more politically influential, profit-driven global corporate agenda for global governance with no explicit requirement for the championing of international human rights. Multilateral trade agreements, such as GATS and TRIPs, have been influential in this process.

A market state can now elect, for example – and many OECD countries have done this – to place 'hospital services' on the 'schedule of commitments' to be covered by the 'liberalising' rules of GATS. This executive action (often no specific parliamentary scrutiny or democratic mandate is necessary) has facilitated a reorganisation of ownership and management of public hospitals on a 'for fee' insurance-oriented model. Under the GATS 'market access' requirement, subsequent (more public goods-minded) governments will be hindered from legislating to regulate the total number or market share of foreign private health care services or suppliers.

The GATS rule of 'national treatment' requires that such a 'liberalising' government cannot provide, even unintentionally, more favourable conditions to domestic health care companies than to foreign corporations. The Most Favored Nation (MFN) rule obligates such administrations to also ensure that most favourable treatment, in terms of trade, granted to any foreign company is extended to all foreign companies wishing to enter this 'liberalised' sector. The 'domestic regulation' rule likewise makes domestic laws and regulations, including those which protect the public's health and safety, subject to challenge and possible elimination if they are determined to be 'unnecessary barriers' to trade, or more 'burdensome than necessary' to assure the quality of a service.

These changes initially facilitate a brief influx of foreign venture capital, but create a one-way policy agenda towards global privatisation of health care services and access to medicines (disadvantaging the frail elderly and disabled, as well as the poor).

In the age of the market state, bilateral preferential trade agreements have also facilitated the plans of multinational pharmaceutical and managed care corporations to exploit 'liberalised' markets and challenge universalist (citizen-funded and egalitarian) domestic health policies, often on the grounds that they have created non-tariff trade barriers, or have insufficiently rewarded 'innovation' or 'research and development'. By threatening to invoke trade sanctions under such agreements, global corporate actors have been able to both exert pressure for positive policy change and build the kind of walls necessary to protect their financial interests from many of the restrictions governments previously imposed in the name of fulfilling foundational social and professional virtues such as justice and respect for human dignity. Public interest 'restrictions' that might be so leveraged include regulations concerned with quarantine, food labelling, safety of the blood supply, access to essential medicines and provision of taxpayer-funded health care in emergencies.

Beyond the age of the market state, however, accumulating credible data is likely to be recognised as proving that the fully privatised health care system such corporate interests and the WTO were promoting failed to reduce, and in fact even exacerbated, the global burden of disease. If so, it will no longer be acceptable in health policy debates to rationalise widespread deaths amongst increasing numbers of poor, uninsured patients and those who cannot get access to essential medicines (because of fiercely protected patents or lack of corporate R&D interest in that area) as temporary market failures or 'adjustments'.[6] The corporate sector will be encouraged by restructured markets to invest in programs that explore alternatives to patents and private insurance as means of promoting socially valuable innovation in health technology and procedures. Increasing numbers of the original policy architects of globally privatised health care are likely to suggest, in such circumstances, an alteration to WTO rules to allow a return to universal (taxpayer-funded and egalitarian) models without having to pay compensation to corporate actors.

II. The role of the pharmaceutical and medical device industries

§i. Problems with 'fast-track' regulatory approvals

In the era of the market state, it is no surprise to see health consumer advocacy organisations privately enlisting executives from pharmaceutical companies such as Eli Lilly & Co. to chart their growth strategies and write their slogans, as well as lobbying policy-makers and safety regulators, to approve treatment programs or products that increase the profits of their drug company donors.

Having the drug and medical device regulators for safety, efficacy, quality and cost-effectiveness fully funded by the industry they are supervising has become an acceptable marketing strategy. The corporate aim here appears to be to create a client-type relationship with regulators. This has tended to decrease the number of warning letters, diminish seizures of mislabelled, defective or dangerous health products, allow more senior management overruling of investigators' enforcement recommendations, promote more 'fast-track' approvals and reduce enforcement actions despite proven problems.

There are substantial risks, however, in pushing corporate influence over regulators too far. For one, falls in investor confidence and stock exchange share price, as well as bankruptcy, become more likely upon announcement in the mass media of any substantial failure in 'fast-tracked' safety regulation of a health care product. Once corporate lobbyists have convinced the state to shift its equity concerns so that it is considered normal to outsource safety regulation of new health technologies, industry is likely to begin to lobby for increased competition amongst such privatised regulators, as is required in other areas of the economy. Why, the argument goes, should an essentially privatised organisation such as the FDA (Federal Drug Administration) have a monopoly over such regulation in the United States, or any other nation?

Beyond the era of the market state, leaders of medical professionalism are likely to more successful in arguing to their colleagues in corporate management, health policy and health technology regulation that taxpayer funding of such regulators will better ensure the arm's-length objectivity required to protect the public.

As humanity strives to emerge from a period where elected representatives tried to convince citizens that citizens' interests were somehow synonymous with those of multinational corporations, leaders amongst health professionals will seek innovative ways to encourage or require the global business world to develop treatments for diseases afflicting poor people in the developing world. Examples are likely to include R&D prize funds for developing treatments for African trypanosomiasis, or leishmaniasis, helminthic infections, schistosomiasis, onchocerciasis, Chagas' disease, malaria, tuberculosis, avian influenza and other emergent infectious diseases. It will be vital for the success of such global pharmaceutical initiatives that they are linked to a robust mechanism for systematically evaluating safety, efficacy, quality and cost-effectiveness before the new products are made widely available to patients.

For even when the governments of developing nations are able to set up drug price reimbursement schemes (in which expert cost-effectiveness evaluation is linked with central government price negotiations) and tender to buy such new drugs at prices close to their international reference price, corruption, counterfeiting, taxes, duties and high mark-ups by dispensing doctors and pharmacies may result in prohibitively high medicine prices for patients. Similarly, these same countries may resent donating emergent infectious disease samples to the WHO, only to see that organisation pass them on to a developed nation corporation that will 'fast-track' develop and patent a treatment that is beyond the budget of most developing countries and their citizens. Such a developing nation may then enter its own arrangement with a corporate multinational to develop a therapy.

Beyond the age of the market state, officials involved in 'fast-track' safety and cost-effectiveness assessments of new health technologies (funded by the public purse and operating within an 'integrated' system of professional regulation) will be less likely to accept placebo-controlled trials and surrogate biomarkers, rather than good evidence of actual health outcomes (such as quality-adjusted life-years). They also will be less likely to disregard the precautionary principle and categorise, for example, new nanotherapeutic products as safe because earlier studies had reached that conclusion about bulk scale equivalents. They will have greater institutional support in resisting the efforts of the pharmaceutical industry to gain approvals through advertising, lobbying, gifts, honoraria and program sponsorships. They will challenge the minimisation of whistleblower protections and any reduction in the capacity of investigative reporting to influence perhaps the strongest sanction in the privatised world of health product development: shareholder confidence.

§ii. 'Innovation's' global assault on cost–effectiveness regulation

In 2003, Abbott Laboratories' anti-AIDS drug Kaletra had global sales of over $1 billion a year. Yet an older and cheaper Abbott AIDS drug called Norvir was a key part of drug regimens that included rival companies' products. Abbott executives (no doubt feeling sufficiently unrestrained by either virtue or legal-based components of regulation) planned to diminish the market value of Norvir, regardless of that drug's comparative safety, efficacy or cost-effectiveness, with the goal of forcing consumers to purchase the more expensive Kaletra.[7] Tactics they contemplated included removing Norvir from the US market, marketing the medicine only in an unpalatable liquid formulation, and ceasing to sell Norvir altogether. They decided to quintuple Norvir's price. The strategy did boost Kaletra sales, and the executives probably assumed that any controversy would eventually fade away.

In 2006, UK-based GlaxoSmithKline (GSK), one of the world's largest (and on some measures most ethical) pharmaceutical companies, announced that it would repay US$3.4 billion to the US Internal Revenue Service (IRS) to settle a 'transfer pricing' dispute involving the shifting of profits between its US and UK subsidiaries.

Merck, another multinational pharmaceutical corporate has four similar tax disputes in the United States and Canada, with potential liabilities of US$5.6 billion. According to the Canada Revenue Agency, Merck transferred patents for several 'blockbuster' drugs to a subsidiary in the low-tax State of Bermuda (Ireland and Puerto Rico have similar industry-friendly policies). Merck then paid that subsidiary artificially inflated amounts for use of the patents, in order to reduce recorded profits. This is possible partly because the real cost of manufacturing brand-name allegedly 'innovative' pharmaceuticals is only approximately 5 per cent of the selling price, and there is no consistent obligation to disclose all details relevant to the marginal cost of production to drug cost-effectiveness regulators.

In Australia in July 2006, the multinational pharmaceutical company Roche was accused of breaching the pharmaceutical industry's self-regulatory code of conduct by spending more than $65,000 taking about 200 top cancer specialists to dinner at exclusive restaurants and paying some to attend overseas marketing events. This code, administered by the industry body Medicines Australia, requires company-sponsored meals to be 'simple and modest'. Roche, based in Switzerland, had annual sales in the preceding year of US$37 billion (greater than the individual GDPs of over 100 small nations), and profits of $7 billion. Global sales of its expensive anti-cancer drugs, including Herceptin (for breast cancer) and MabThera (for non-Hodgkins lymphoma), rose 42 per cent between 2004 and 2006. It was around this time that Herceptin was finally (after multiple prior submissions) listed on Australia's Pharmaceutical Benefits Scheme (PBS) for government reimbursement after expert cost-effectiveness evaluation.[8] There was concern that such largesse could appear to be a reward for the pressure such doctors had exerted to have Roche drugs listed on the PBS, or that Australian specialists, due to their excellent clinical reputation, were perceived by the company as making good potential international marketing agents.

Cost-effectiveness analysis of medicines, directly or indirectly challenged in the above examples, represents, in most European nations, Australia, Canada and New Zealand, a fourth hurdle (after quality, safety and efficacy regulatory evaluation) to be overcome by a medicines manufacturer prior to marketing. In the age beyond the market state, it will become an increasingly prominent part of all health care systems, regardless of their prior level of privatisation.

In the age of the market state, cost-effectiveness analysis has remained a subdued component of the influential, and substantially privatised, US health care system. It largely takes place there through covert negotiations between drug manufacturers, state Medicaid officers, HMO officials and committees at individual hospitals, as well as in specialised departments such as Veterans' Affairs. Industry, however, has successfully lobbied against the capacity of the US federal government to link its potential monopsony (sole purchaser) buying power with cost-effectiveness analysis of both medicines and medical devices through a positive list reimbursement scheme assisted, for example, by the US Agency for Health care Research and Quality (AHRQ).[9]

Pharmaceutical companies generally have not minded cost-effectiveness analysis of their new products being carried out by expert purchasing committees at individual health care institutions, as those committees have had only limited leverage in price negotiations. Such global businesses have also learnt how to manipulate clinical trials to avoid head-to-head comparisons with cheaper competitors, as well as how to maximise (often under-dosed) surrogate outcome measures (such as decreases in blood pressure or cholesterol) instead of quality life-years gained. They have had two main objections to any global enhancement of the process of cost-effectiveness evaluation.

The first objection was to 'reference pricing'. This is a technique in which expert assessors work through a hierarchy of evidence in comparing the value of a pharmaceutical recently approved (on quality, safety and efficacy grounds) on its core clinical indication against already marketed therapies of the same therapeutic class (for example anti-depressants, anti-hypertensives, lipid-lowering or anti-asthma medications). If the new drug is shown to be not truly 'innovative' (that is, not more cost-effective than existing products in that therapeutic class), its price is 'referenced' thereafter to the average or lowest in that class. This technique is one of the few policy levers that draws the taxpayer (government-funded) reimbursement level for new branded drugs towards an equilibrium where equivalent prices are achieved for similarly performing drugs. It avoids market failure by encouraging whole industry competition, allowing generic manufacturers to sustain a reasonably high (but not excessive) return, and being consistent with regulatory schemes that facilitate global mass marketed super low cost generics and closed bid tenders (which give a better indication of marginal cost of production).

In the age of the market state, however, the representatives of brand-name, so-called innovative pharmaceutical manufacturers (including the US Trade Representative [USTR]) have vigorously opposed reference pricing in lobbying discussions with government Health Ministers. They have argued that reference pricing somehow opposes 'innovation', which key bilateral trade agreements (though not defining it) require to be rewarded on pain of trade sanctions. They lobby those Ministers for policies that give 'head room' in government reimbursement schemes to new and allegedly 'innovative' drugs by making mandatory price reductions in generic products.

Their second and main objection, however, has been to the process of evaluating pharmaceutical 'innovation' through expert scientific evidence-based analysis of objectively demonstrated therapeutic significance, particularly when this is linked to a central government price negotiation. These concerns were exemplified in industry lobbying taking place in conjunction with negotiations around the Australia–US Free Trade Agreement (AUSFTA) and the South Korea–US Free Trade Agreement (KORUSFTA).

The AUSFTA, for example, required discussions between the US FDA and the Australian TGA (Therapeutic Drugs Administration) about making 'innovative' pharmaceutical products more speedily available (Annex 2C.4) and the facilitation of greater regulatory recognition of pharmaceutical 'innovation'. It also provided an ambiguous definition of pharmaceutical 'innovation' that allowed it to be determined by either the operation of a 'competitive market' (the US approach) or by 'objectively demonstrated therapeutic significance' (the Australian method) (Annex 2C.1).[10]

The Korean negotiators to the KORUSFTA, previously briefed by the author on the content and process behind the AUSFTA medicines provisions, opened negotiations in this area with a demand to be allowed to establish a PBS-style positive list cost-effectiveness evaluation system linked to central government price negotiation. They were also encouraged to insert in the relevant KORUSFTA provision a vaguely defined reference to 'objectively demonstrated therapeutic value' to balance the deliberately uncertain meaning of the term 'innovation' and allow greater parity in subsequent policy discussion.

Another important tactic of pharmaceutical multinationals has involved 'evergreening'. 'Evergreening' is prolonging the legally enforceable life of any one of the numerous patents (relating to new uses or delivery systems, for instance) that cluster around the soon-to-expire active therapeutic ingredient patent for a blockbuster brand-name pharmaceutical. 'Evergreening' strategies include simply 'buying off' a generic company so that it cannot launch a competitor product, creating licensing agreements so that generics are 'authorised' by brand-name companies, patenting minor molecular variations to patent-expiring 'blockbuster' products, and merely patenting the placement of the patent-expiring drug in pill combination with another.

Some bilateral trade agreements also have TRIPs-minus provisions increasing the period of data exclusivity (when a generic manufacturer can't get access to the initial clinical trial data). This might not only inhibit compulsory licensing; if put together with multiple uses, it could inhibit indefinitely preparation by a generic manufacturer for 'springboarding' upon patent expiry. It could also facilitate brand-name industry claims that such 'springboarding' represents a loss of profits from their investment in producing the original data.

Such arguments are in clear opposition to the accepted social contract idea that intellectual property rights (more accurately termed intellectual monopoly privileges [IMPs]) are really only a temporary monopoly (not a natural right) granted by the community in return for the public benefit of rapidly disseminated knowledge.

Of most concern, however, in the 'evergreening' department, will be the requirement inserted in NAFTA (the North American Free Trade Agreement, which involves the United States, Canada and Mexico), the AUSFTA and probably KORUSFTA that regulatory quality, efficacy and safety approval not be given for a generic drug until a 'linked' check has been made by the same medicines regulator that no patents are being infringed. Canada got around the worst excesses of this 'linkage' system by creating a specialised agency (the Office of Patented Medicines and Liaison) to investigate patent claims over new therapeutic products and determine whether those claims were only invalid 'me-too' (non-innovative) or 'evergreening' ones.

Major European and US pharmaceutical and biotechnology industry associations have similarly not only sought to drive the industry lobbying principle of 'innovation' into the cost-effectiveness systems of OECD regulators, but also lobbied for 'reforms' that appear to be merely technical adjustments, but whose real goal is to facilitate commercial advantage. One example involves the WHO adopting a policy of granting unique International Nonproprietary Names (INNs) to each biopharmaceutical product from every company, rather than generic names based on the active agent. Such a change, though seeming an insignificant technical adjustment, would make it harder for physicians and health policy-makers to allow generic substitution in prescriptions.

Another significant component of the global marketing strategy of pharmaceutical multinationals has involved facilitating the spread in health policy of support for so-called direct-to-consumer advertising. This is a process that essentially creates an apparently unimpeded but in fact distorted information flow between a manufacturer and health product consumers. It undercuts conceptions of competence and standard of care associated with medical professionals as learned intermediaries. As well as being facilitated by free trade agreements (for example, Annex 2C.5 of the AUSFTA), it has been assisted by many other industry strategies. CanWest Global Communications, for example, challenged a Canadian Federal law that bans US-style 'direct-to-consumer' advertisements for prescription drugs. CanWest claimed that the current Canadian law restricted its freedom of expression under the Canadian Charter of Rights and freedoms, and that it was being denied the ability to earn advertising revenue like its US counterparts.

This raised the broader issue of whether corporations, being artificial persons, should be allowed, beyond the age of the market state, to rely on human rights protections. If corporate and government interests have merged in a market state arrangement, international law needs to allow such corporations to also be found liable for failing to protect, respect and fulfil international human rights. 'Integrated' regulation could be considered to have really begun to work once health care corporations are able to exercise a conscience in the public good, become, in effect, married and support a family, vote and take on other community responsibilities. These would indicate that they are striving to achieve virtues by the consistent application of universally applicable principles in the face of obstacles, for example by focusing on sustainability and achievement of some UN Millennium Development Goals to ameliorate their addiction to ever-increasing profits. Perhaps only at that point should they be presumptively accorded the core international right to respect for their intrinsic human dignity.

Beyond the era of the market state, if cost-effectiveness regulators try to implement policies that rein in the prices of 'innovative' medicines and medical devices, their corporate manufacturers will have less capacity to threaten Ministers with taking their business and related investments elsewhere. They will likewise have reduced ability (as a result of constitutional and legislative reforms) to leverage favourable policy outcomes by offering post-public office employment to bureaucratic staff willing to run a pro-industry agenda.

Further, such an agenda would be influenced by the enhanced integration of corporate executives and health policy-makers into a regulatory system promoting foundational social and professional virtues and principles. As a result, it may be less likely to involve, for example, socially divisive chiefly pro-industry policy recommendations such as the undercutting of reference pricing, the 'fast-tracking' of regulatory approvals in practical circumvention of the precautionary principle, the gradual replacement of centralised cost-effectiveness schemes, and the creation of uncapped government subsidies (for example, a percentage of whatever cost consumers are asked to bear) of private health and medicines insurance, or even health care and medicines savings accounts.

§iii. Public-funded research and renewal in the biopharma industry

Shakespeare's *The Tempest* opens, as many doctor–patient relationships also do, with a cataclysmic storm producing much human suffering. As in *King Lear*, this upheaval in the elements may be interpreted as symbolic of tumult in the moral world. But like the contemporary hurricanes whose destructiveness is enhanced by global warming, *The Tempest*'s storm is produced by man himself. Prospero, with resonances to Leonardo da Vinci and Christopher Marlowe's Dr Faustus, had previously dedicated himself to developing virtue amongst his community. Now, betrayed into exile, this storm and the knowledge acquired from 'magic' books (the analogy particularly suggesting modern medical research in genetic manipulation and nanotechnology), by allowing his will to become sovereign, give him the opportunity to either profit from and exacerbate, or relieve, the suffering of a number of people.

Encouraging a strong biotechnology sector will be a central component of health and industry policy beyond the age of the market state. Nations are more likely to reap direct rewards (through taxation) or indirect benefits (via improved population health outcomes) if biotechnology companies gain adequate capitalisation to move therapeutics to the clinical trial stage. To do this they will still need to acquire intellectual monopoly privileges through patents, secure leading scientists and 'name' directors, and attract 'seed' (or 'venture') as well as more 'patient' capital.

To help them consistently maintain share price, governments should continue, by various forms of regulation, to facilitate low-taxation clusters (in close geographical proximity) or more virtual collaborations with public and private R&D organisations. One significant difference, however, will be that the leaders of such corporations and governments will be more consistently focused on ensuring that their respective efforts endorse foundational social and professional virtues. Health technology corporations and their staff will actively promote their different roles and responsibilities (now no longer purely financial) to shareholders and to the wider community.

Beyond the age of the market state, an 'integrated' professional regulatory system will facilitate transparent institutional processes whereby demands by safety and cost-effectiveness assessors for head-to-head randomised control trials (RCTs) can be objectively weighed against, for example, industry interest in using placebos (because this allegedly expedites regulatory approval and rarely causes 'serious harm') or provisional regulatory marketing approval with post-marketing surveillance utilising pharmacogenomics (including genetic tests before drug prescription).

Research and clinical ethics committees properly funded and protected with statutory immunity in accordance with international standards will carefully scrutinise clinical trials amongst the world's impoverished or destitute sick. Medical journals publishing the results of such RCTs (the gold standard of the 'evidence-based medicine' movement) will be more likely to mandate reporting on the research subjects' understanding and giving or refusing of informed consent, on researchers' conflicts of interest, on the use of inducements or coercion, and even on whether an information sheet had been provided. It will no longer be acceptable to simply add a single non-transparent line or paragraph to a publication stating that the study had been approved by some ethics committee.[11]

One future scenario is for an increasingly 'closed' research culture in which secrecy, patents, commercial-in-confidence arrangements and dependence of the private sector for research funding supplant collegiality and the sharing of knowledge for the benefit of individual patients and the public. An alternative, however, involves the proliferation of science commons, patent pools, open-source initiatives, clearing house mechanisms and collective rights arrangements. The latter are more likely to sustain public confidence, draw in high-quality researchers and encourage investor confidence in eventual but prolonged dividends. They are also more likely to be coherent with traditional conceptions of medical professionalism.

§iv. *Biopharma techno-garden or nanotech fortress world?*

In Jorge Luis Borges' story *Tlön, Uqbar, Orbis Tertius*, two friends are described as finding, at the conclusion of an old cyclopaedia, an article on a hitherto unknown country called Uqbar and, later, a volume about its world, the *First Encyclopaedia of Tlön*. Imagine Uqbar and Tlön to be the names of a hypothetical country and the earth itself, in the age that begins to supersede that of the market state.

By this time, humans may have created a planetary civilisation, perhaps even with the capacity to travel intergalactically, for example, by shrinking space faster than the speed of light, or to other universes by sending themselves, as information, through a 'wormhole' (Kerr rotating black holes or Einstein-Rosen bridges), building a star system atom smasher, or compressing a tiny amount of matter to enormous energies and densities.[12] The big issue is not whether such achievements are technologically possible, but if humanity will evolve rapidly enough morally to sustain itself during their development.

Consider, for example, the difficulties for a health professional seeking virtue through dedicated performance of his or her professional responsibilities when patented genetic engineering and nanotechnology has allowed privately insured patients' skin to be made regionally transparent at will (say, to assist diagnosis); or blood to combine on self-command outside the body into storable or disposable packages (to assist trauma resuscitation). What if nanocomputers were able to lock onto individual red or white blood cells, analyse their functioning and inject appropriate treatments, or nanoneuro implants allow memory to rapidly store and recall vast amounts of complex knowledge?

People living in such a 'techno-garden' reality may come to resent the need to have a knowledge elite (such as health professionals) controlling any aspect of their lives. Will health professionals, to the extent that they do exist then as a separate group, and the society that supports them, resent the fact that millions of children continue to die every year from lack of food or clean water, or from warfare, particularly when disease or illness should be a very rare and readily self-repairable event universally (not just amongst the wealthy)?

Will they support an 'adaptive-mosaic' vision of the future (involving small sustainable communities emphasising high-valued intermediate technologies and micro-credit in lifestyle-rich rural areas competing with low-priced more standardised goods from the global marketplace in large urban locations)?

Perhaps instead of such an 'integrated' market facilitating lifestyle competition, expert oligarchies will organise a 'fortress world', or 'global orchestration' modes of existence. Two seeds for such future choices, increased human genome knowledge and nanotechnology, have already been sown.

The Human Genome Project (HGP) was commenced in 1988 and finally announced as completed on 14 April 2003 – by an International Genome Sequencing Consortium led in the United States but involving significant contributions from most developed nations. Finalisation of the HGP was a close-run contest between the public (Sulston) and private (Venter) sectors, the latter prepared to close out community access to the new knowledge to foster 'innovation' through profit-earning patent rights.

As a result of the HGP, the 750 megabytes of information about each of the approximately 30,000 genes in each human body may eventually be stored in databases and ultimately in desktop computers. The HGP was often described as a scientific revolution likely to provide new 'maps' that would redraw many ethical, legal and human rights boundaries for humanity: 5 per cent of the overall HGP budget was dedicated to studying related ethical, legal and social issues (ELSI).

The ultimate usefulness of the HGP was often presented to the public in terms of the medical profession being able to eventually triumph over human disease and even the ageing process. The final information represented an average of all the DNA samples involved, not the DNA of any particular individual, nationality or racial group. It is not surprising, then, that international regulatory efforts should have been made to recognise the human genome, like the sea bed, the moon or outer space, or our great cultural and natural treasures, as part of the 'common heritage of humanity'.

Corporate use of HGP-derived knowledge may impact on medical professionalism through redefinitions of core duty-defining concepts such as 'patient'. Patients certainly traditionally did not include clones, chimeras, genetically modified embryos, animals, the environment, future generations, the genetically at-risk 'worried well', or relatives of someone with a genetic predisposition to disease, or those with some socially or individually undesirable trait. These difficulties for medical professionalism will be compounded if strong artificial intelligence is perfected and nanocomputers with human-like genotypes come to assert that they have self-consciousness equal, if not superior, to ours.

Likewise problematic will be the terms 'disease' (is an asymptomatic 'carrier' of an abnormal gene diseased?), 'normality' (who defines the 'normal' human genome?) and 'personal responsibility' (should criminal conduct be punished if genes seemingly dictate it?). Most diseases are experienced as ego-alien, externalised threats. Genetic disorders, however, cannot be as readily projected outwards psychologically.

Medical nanotechnology, another factor in future health policy decisions, involves the development of drug/invasive therapeutic device products controllable at atomic, molecular or macromolecular levels of approximately 1–100 nanometers, a nanometer being one-billionth of a metre. It is a rapidly expanding area of medical research globally, with revolutionary implications for diagnosis and treatment.

The research budget of every major pharmaceutical company now has a considerable component devoted to nanotechnology. Peptide nanotubes, for example, have been investigated as the next generation of antibiotics and as immune modulators. Nanogenerators that use an antibody to direct a caged radioactive atom to destroy cancer cells are being engineered. Nanoparticles may provide an efficient delivery system for DNA vaccines and gene therapy. They may allow speedier and more efficient delivery of drugs to diseased cells, with less pain. They are already being investigated for use in neurosurgery, cardiac surgery and blood disorders.

In 2005, the US FDA announced approval for a silver nanotechnology coating that purports to render common invasive medical devices relatively impervious to infection-causing bacteria. Nanotechnology products appear to be 'innovative' (at least on the vague brand-name industry definition). But their safety, quality and efficacy regulatory approval may be based on prior assessment of bulk-scale materials, ignoring the precautionary principle.

This should be a matter of concern for medical professionalism, because nanoparticles are highly reactive and mobile within the human body, and so present unique and largely unexplored health risks. Nanoparticles accumulate chiefly in the mitochondria, producing free radicals and cell damage. Yet nanoparticulate 'clear' sunscreens have been approved by safety regulators because of a lack of evidence that they are capable of passing through the dead cells of the outer skin. This conclusion seems inconsistent with the considerable research being done on using nanotechnology to facilitate transcutaneous vaccination and with the common sense understanding that many people using such nanosunscreens will have cuts, abrasions and excoriating skin conditions such as eczema. There are currently no effective methods of monitoring nanoparticle exposure risks in patients or health care workers. A probable long disease latency period after exposure to nanoparticles – as was the case with asbestosis and silicosis – means that causation will be difficult to prove legally and compensation will therefore be difficult to obtain. In the post-market state era, complying with the precautionary principle is more likely to be a dominant regulatory concern than is ensuring that the share price of nanotechnology companies remains unchallenged.

Also, nanomedical products are likely to be ubiquitous and highly priced components of a future health care system. They will probably be linked to stronger cost-effectiveness claims related to rewarding 'innovation' than were made for traditional medicines and medical devices. This points to the public benefit of cost-effectiveness assessments of 'innovative' health technology products being accepted as a routine fourth hurdle to marketing approval, after safety, efficacy and quality evaluation.

Genetic research appears to be showing that DNA is both extremely similar amongst all life forms and interchangeable. As our understanding of other species (including their capacity to suffer) broadens, our sympathy and capacity to ascribe to such life forms 'interests' capable of protection by ethical and legal principles will also expand. The intuitive convictions and emotional responses generated by 'human dignity' are not qualitatively different from those many people feel towards animals or ecosystems. James Lovelock, for example, promoted 'geophysiology' as the name for the skills needed by a physician to treat the sick and damaged Earth as a self-sustaining natural system – now best imagined as a patient (called Gaia).[13]

In the post-market state era, will leaders amongst medical professionals acknowledge that we should show other species equal concern and respect within a global community of principle (say, to protect them from extinction, regardless of the 'interests' they may or may not possess), even if our legal system does not designate them 'persons' or 'patients'? Related challenges for professional leaders will include regulatory responses to climate change, access to scarce water, genetically modified crops, patented seeds, sanitation and pollution (perhaps using nanotechnology and biotechnologically developed organisms able to contain harmful emissions and chemicals).

§v. Enclosing, or sharing, techno-garden fruits of knowledge

In Peter Goldsworthy's novel *Honk if You Are Jesus*, a wealthy research institute obtains reputedly genuine relics of Christ. The plan of the institute's board is to reproduce the historical Jesus by *in vitro* nuclear transfer of his DNA into an oocyte thence implanted in a virgin bride. Such an outlandish scheme illustrates, at its most extreme, a philosophy known as genetic reductionism. Genetic reductionism, in the ontological sense, claims that a patient's consciousness, conscience, emotions, soul or even free will, must ultimately be related to genetic structure or be said not to exist.

In the future, somatic and germ-line gene therapy, biobanks and stem cell research offer the possibility of detecting, preventing and regenerating diseased organs. This could eliminate the need for anti-rejection immune suppressant medication. A major issue for medical professionalism will be how to make such advances in medical technology available to all citizens. Patents (intellectual monopoly privileges) may enclose this knowledge so that it makes excessive corporate profits, and as a result is available only to those wealthy enough to afford private health insurance.

Related health policy questions concern whether gene-based medicine should be subsidised in the role of, or allowed to be advertised by corporate patent-holders as, a 'social equaliser'. The pressure to competently and compassionately deal with the resultant genetic reductionist expectations, particularly for poor people, will be a significant burden on health professionals loyal to relief of patient suffering as the age of the market state draws to a close.

The 'pool' of taxpayer-created funds available to the state for the fulfilment of its responsibilities with regard to health care can be viewed as a contemporary equivalent of a medieval agricultural 'common'.[14] In this context, patents over the human genome, plus medical procedures (or processes) and new health technologies (including pharmaceuticals and medical devices), may be considered part of a globalised enclosure movement.

The patenting of medical knowledge in the form of procedures or processes, for example, has been unsuccessfully opposed by the medical profession (for example in the 2006 *LabCorp Case* before the US Supreme Court) as fundamentally contradicting professional responsibilities that prioritise loyalty to the relief of patient suffering. Similarly, patents have been taken out over the ('junk') stretches of DNA that may be involved in genetic tests. If such tests become a ubiquitous part of the standard of care before diagnosis, or before administration of a drug (pharmacogenomcs), that will significantly raise costs within, and challenge the social and professional values of, any substantially privatised health care system.

One particular area of controversy may concern whether such patents should restrict a putative right to be born healthy (that is, by use of pre-implantation or intra-utero gene therapy). Some courts have already referred to 'the fundamental right of a child to be born as a whole, functional human being',[15] or the 'right to begin life with a sound mind and body'.[16]

In an 'integrated' system of professional regulation such an inchoate principle may be calibrated by decision-makers against accepted bioethical and constitutional privacy protections, the international human rights of the disabled to life, to reproduce, to be free from cruel or degrading treatment and to bodily integrity, as well as the state's general legal responsibility to protect vulnerable citizens, including unborn children. An assertion of a 'right' of an adult 'consumer' to be assured a minimum level of health, which is fraught with problems for personal responsibility and community duty, would appear somewhat less coherent under such a process.

In the age beyond the market state, intellectual monopoly privilege provisions in the WTO TRIPs agreement and in bilateral trade agreements will be less likely to allow enhanced patent terms to restrict access to existing and future medicines and medical technology. This will be partly because there is more likely to be a consensus amongst the relevant knowledge elites that excessively concentrated corporate ownership and control of information, technology, biological resources and culture will only foster growing inequality of access to education, knowledge and technology, and thus undermine not only growth of freedom, democracy and social cohesion, but industry sustainability.

With development of a global regulatory system that better correlates research and development with global burden of disease, there will be less need for pharmaceutical multinationals such as Merck, Pfizer and Eli Lilly to claim that generic drug manufacturers (the ones they have not bought out, licensed or controlled by other business and regulatory tactics), particularly in developing nations, are modern-day 'pirates' who are stealing their intellectual capital. There will be a greater amount of scientific evidence available by which to judge the truth of industry claims that TRIPs gives the same global patent protection to developing and developed countries, and that allowing largely unrestricted access by corporate multinationals to domestic economies will help developing countries get richer so that they can afford 'fair' prices for drugs and stop 'free-riding' on the putative global public good of US research and development.

Global health policy development, in other words, will become more evidence-based, rather than ideology-based. Beyond the age of the market state it will be unacceptable, under an 'integrated' system of professional regulation, for a panel of three trade lawyers to have the final say on whether or not a multilateral or bilateral trade agreement requires changes to domestic public health legislation solely because the latter is non-compliant with TRIPs.[17]

Finally, beyond the age of the market state, 'integrated' global regulatory processes will be more likely to support the position that patents over the human genome, essential medicines and life-saving medical processes should be policed to ensure that they do not contravene bioethical and human rights principles requiring communal 'solidarity', respect for the foundational virtue of human dignity, and benefit-sharing. Likewise, they should support the proposition that the human genome is the common heritage of humanity and should thus be held in trust as a product of the natural world over which man is steward.

§vi. Medical 'gatekeeping': Genetic and nano surveillance in a fortress world

The World State in Aldous Huxley's *Brave New World* promotes its programs and policies under the motto 'Community, Identity, Stability'. In large grey skyscrapers, embryos are artificially 'hatched' *ex utero* and later 'conditioned' by the state to contentedly perform chosen tasks in society. Babies of the khaki-clad genetic Delta caste, for example, are exposed to repetitive loud noises and mild electric shocks to condition them against liking poetry books or flowers. In such a world, people do not develop virtue, for they have no temptations, no vices to struggle against. Their conditioned personalities have few inclinations or opportunities to be compassionate, noble or heroic. If strong intuitive convictions do arise, say about disloyalty or injustice, such unstable emotions can be easily calmed by consuming two or three half-gram tablets of the drug *soma*.

Huxley's fictional world represents a totalitarian extreme, but medical professionalism is moving into a future with very real threats that the market state will use genetic information (with the assistance of nanotechnology) to reshape its own priorities: staying in political power and ensuring the continuance of very large profits for multinational corporate sponsors and friends. In such an environment, disclosure of genetic information (even for apparently therapeutically valid reasons related to individual or public health) could have extremely deleterious consequences for a patient.

A fully privatised global health care system is likely to be based on the private insurance model, and may involve closely related concepts such as health and/or medicines savings accounts. An insurance contract creates a legal relationship of *uberrima fides*, requiring full disclosure of information relevant to risk selection, classification, and underwriting. On the basis of information provided by insurees, insurers determine what level of contribution each policyholder should make to the common pool which is distributed to those who die (life insurance), become disabled (disability insurance) or develop illness (health insurance). Most insurance policies exclude treatment for pre-existing conditions, and there is a real concern that genetic screening or testing which reveals an abnormality may trigger this exclusion. Expenses for prophylactic treatments based on genetic predispositions might also not be covered. In such circumstances, doctors sensitive to their professional responsibilities will need to calibrate legislation that reduces, for example, public funding or private insurance cover for the disabled, or implies that parents who knowingly carry a genetically 'abnormal' fetus to term are irresponsible, against norms of bioethics and international human rights.

Pre and post-employment genetic testing likewise will become more frequent, as the sensitivity, specificity of, and patent royalties from such investigations improve and greater knowledge is gained about the health risks of exposing certain genotypes to particular workplace environments. As far back as the 1970s, for instance, the

DuPont corporation in the United States began genetic screening for a trait that could predispose to sickle cell anaemia when those so affected were exposed to certain environmental stresses (such as diminution of environmental oxygen). This was ostensibly for the 'information and edification' of employees, but doctors hired by the company nonetheless had to explain why some people so tested were subsequently not hired.

Medical participation in workplace genetic testing appears to satisfy the primary social and professional virtues in respect of the public benefits of early disease detection. The capacity of the same information to promote social discrimination and stigmatisation, however, will set challenges for medical professionals in terms of respecting patient confidentiality and preventing or ameliorating discriminatory employer decisions based on misconceptions about such results. Many genetic abnormalities will continue to arise from unpredictable mutations. Even if a disease is accurately predicted, its expression as symptoms, and its severity, time of onset and susceptibility to treatment, may vary enormously. A further pressure may arise from the trend to outsource employee medical services, removing occupational physicians to off-site positions, relying on less expensive nursing and paramedical care in the first instance.

Doctors, finally, will have an important role as gatekeepers for the entry of DNA, or its related genetic information, into the criminal justice system. Legislation expressly authorising forensic DNA sampling will be far from uniform in requiring that specimens be taken in a hospital or medical facility, or even by a physician. Where legislative provisions allowing search, and the obtaining of identifying particulars, do not expressly include the power to obtain a genetic sample, the power to order a medical examination may become a *de facto* means to the same end. Doctors who perform such tests may face additional dilemmas: about adequately communicating the resultant information to patients and about notifying others, such as spouses or relatives, who may not wish to know, but could be endangered if they do not.

III. Promoting global public goods in health care

As key promoters of the globalisation of their own nation's model of privatised health care, US officials have been scrupulous in attempting to limit the creation of norms (or principles) promoting global public goods.

Early in 2006, for example, US officials visited the WHO director-general in Geneva to discuss that organisation's Thailand representative. That WHO employee had recently published an opinion-editorial piece warning that the US–Thai Free Trade Agreement (THAIUSFTA) negotiations would restrict Thailand's sovereign rights to invoke *Doha Declaration*-supported TRIPs public interest exceptions to pharmaceutical intellectual property rights. The alleged consequence was probable bankruptcy for Thailand's 30 baht universal health care scheme. Soon afterwards that WHO official was transferred to another country.[18] After a changed Thai government decided to issue a compulsory licence to make cheaper copies of a Merck-produced anti-HIV/AIDS drug, US officials (and the WHO) actively opposed aspects of that TRIPs-justified action too.

In a world where domestic markets are opened to global trade, local economies are also exquisitely vulnerable to trade sanctions imposed under international trade agreements. In such circumstances it can readily become a corporate strategy to use threat of such sanctions to ensure that trade deal principles (concerning pharmaceuticals, blood fractionation, or quarantine, for example) lead to appropriate changes in public health legislation. This may represent a form of *de facto* sovereignty over domestic democratic processes and the rule of law that can said to characterise health policy in the era of the market state.

To date, most of the provisions about health matters included in international trade agreements have supported a private rights, multinational corporate agenda. This need not necessarily be so, however, and this section explores some preliminary options that could be debated in any renegotiation of the global social contract aimed at using international trade agreements to drive a global public goods renewal program in health care.

§i. *Private vs public goods in the trade agenda*

The official position of the committee monitoring the *ICESCR* is that privatisation of clinical medicine, though it may affect whether a state's duty is to 'protect' rather than 'respect' human rights, does not, of itself, necessarily adversely interfere with that state's obligation to fulfil public health responsibilities under the human right to health.[19] Yet obligations to protect individuals from third party violations could create state responsibility to protect patients from health care corporations or their employees even where such doctors are not considered state agents; this is one interpretation, for example, of the requirement of 'free consent' in Article 7 of the *ICCPR*.

Beyond the age of the market state, an 'integrated' professional regulatory system will more effectively encourage pharmaceutical multinationals to contribute to the pool of taxpayer funds available to pay for public goods. These public goods will increasingly be defined to include the global accomplishment of government policies and community effort available to be enjoyed by all, not merely consumption that, by technical economic definition, does not detract from use by another.

One mechanism for facilitating this process and making the worldwide health care system more responsive to the global burden of disease, is to ensure that international trade agreements express a better balance between private and public goods. Trade sanctions applicable under such agreements, for example, could be used to drive social agendas related to decarbonisation (shifting from fossil fuel to renewable energy) and dematerialisation (reducing use of unnecessary consumer goods and advertising for them), as well as programs for disability services, universal health care and essential medicines.

Another strategy involves the creation of specific treaties that include provisions facilitating global licensing of multinational corporations, such as taxes payable by such corporations to go to the United Nations, and corporate responsibilities over mutually negotiated specific community or public goods projects. Such proposals would regard corporations by law as people seeking to develop virtue, as they must be if they are to participate more meaningfully in the progression of the better hopes and ideals of humanity as reflected in the principles of the international human rights system. Corporations are more likely to want to do this if such treaties also redefine their responsibilities to shareholders and the training of their chief executives (within an 'integrated' professional regulatory system, for example).

A related policy suggestion is to facilitate economic efficiencies and normative integration by merging the offices, functions and processes of the WTO, the WHO and the Human Rights Council.

These changes, promoting coherence (or what others might call consilience or congruence) between trade and wider human goals, may be assisted by moves to facilitate registration for voting – by individual citizens or communities – on issues before the WTO, the WHO and the United Nations. This may require establishing a new, non state-based constitution for such international organisations.

Other global social contract renegotiation proposals for the post-market state era could involve promoting the role of not-for-profit corporations, professional encouragement of domestic constitutional protections of universal access to health care, particularly in emergencies and to essential medicines, and an experimental use patent exemption for taxpayer-funded university-based researchers. Enhanced protection of whistleblowers from unjust reprisals, and financial (*qui tam*) encouragement for them, may also help facilitate public goods related to safety and cost-effectiveness in this area, as will strong anti-trust laws and pro-competition agencies.

An important component of a new global social contract could be a system for rewarding – with sustainable levels of government reimbursement – medicines and medical device 'innovation' established through internationally harmonised, independent expert assessment of health technology safety, quality, efficacy and cost-effectiveness, funded by a tax on global financial transactions.[20] The treaty creating such a post-market state global regulatory system would list the principles underpinning such assessments: for example, safety, quality, efficacy, equity of access, and a sustainable and responsible industry. This global policy proposal is discussed in greater detail in the next chapter.

§ii. *Financing global public goods to tame health care privatisation*

In the Isaac Asimov story *The Gods Themselves*, a scientist discovers a strange kind of plutonium – plutonium186 – derived from a parallel universe where the nuclear force is much stronger, thus overcoming the repulsion of protons and releasing large amounts of energy. He patents a device to harness this energy, but the device risks exploding the sun, through a general increase in our universe's nuclear force. The corporate sector continues nonetheless to profitably exploit the new energy, despite the dire consequences. They back scientists who support, as a solution, using an atom smasher to create a hole to another universe.

Private ownership of global health care delivery will not create so many difficulties if it is balanced by institutional support for global public goods. Such goods, as mentioned, provide benefits from which no individual is excluded, and span national, cultural and generational boundaries. Support for global public goods in health care seems a logical outcome of a professional regulatory system's foundation on social and professional virtues, as well as the solidification of corporate globalisation and greater empiric evidence of the burden of disease.

Examples of such global public goods include clean air, peaceful societies, control of communicable disease, transport and law and order infrastructure, and systems of universal health care. Some of these require international cooperation for their production (safety and cost-effectiveness evaluation of new health technologies). Developing mechanisms for the policing, administration and joint cooperative financing of global public goods, particularly those in the form of natural and cultural commons (including items designated common heritage of humanity or on the UNESCO World Heritage Lists), may herald the end of the market state era.

Global public goods, at least until universal threats such as terrorism, emergent infectious disease and global warming create sufficient political will for reform of world governance structures, will have to be financed at the national level, with sector-specific incentives. These must recognise country preferences (developing nations may prioritise peace, safe air and water as well as affordable essential medicines and seeds ahead of stability of international financial structures). National policy attention to domestic public health goods – through, for example, carbon emission and energy taxes, pollution control, universal access to health services, improvements in human rights conditions that discourage international flows of asylum seekers, discouragement of terrorism and prevention of corruption – will be more widely recognised as discouraging cross-border 'spillovers' that erode global public goods.[21] Fishing quotas, carbon emission permits, contributions to UN organisations and foreign aid are other examples of global public goods that would benefit from greater financial and administrative cooperation between nations, linked with increased democratic involvement in policy development.

One specific strategy in the health technology field is for public goods-focused researchers to incrementally innovate drug molecules and, by institutionally treating each new patent as a public good, make the product available cheaply to patients in the developing world. English medical researchers, for example, recently redesigned an effective but extremely expensive Roche drug for hepatitis C, called pegylated interferon, so that its large sugar molecule (which increased its half life) is on the inside, rather than the outside. The Shantha corporation in Hyderabad, which had made the world's first cost-effective hepatitis B vaccine (and was already making the original interferon), agreed to make the new medicine with the Indian government subsidising the necessary pre-regulatory approval clinical trials. The UK scientists are also working on a similarly innovative 'ethical pharmaceutical' for visceral leishmaniasis (kala-azar), a disease transmitted by sandflies that is fatal in Brazil, Bangladesh, India and the Sudan.[22]

Finally, a treaty facilitating intranational micro-credit could bring the creativity and innovation of the worlds's poor (with the assistance of social entrepreneurs) into a revitalised and more equitable global health care market. Related global regulatory systems may facilitate genuine competition between health care executives out to amass more personal profit (or for their shareholders) and those seeking venture capital to achieve specific public goods and lifestyle targets. Such progress should not be retarded by policy acquiescence to technical economic definitions of public goods that limit the capacity of social entrepreneurs to integrate market norms with broader human values and aspirations.

Chapter summary and cases for further discussion

- In the age of the market state, the capacity of doctors to relieve patient suffering has been advertised as in large part a measure of the innovation and efficiency of HMOs and health technology manufacturers, in particular those producing expensive new gene-based drugs and nanotherapeutics.

- Global private health care and health technology companies promoted, through their public relations consultants, an image of their organisations as good corporate citizens. But any legislated requirement that such efforts be systematically tracked, compared against competitors, and independently evaluated and publicised, was vigorously resisted.

- The WTO TRIPs and GATS agreements, as well as bilateral trade agreements with health-related provisions, have been significant instruments in the facilitation of the ideological agenda for full privatisation of global health care.

- Beyond the age of the market state, multinational health technology companies will be more willing to allow global regulation through treaties such as that on safety and cost-effectiveness expert assessment of new health technologies.

- Health professionals will continue to play important regulatory roles in 'gatekeeping' the entry of patient genetic data into private employment, insurance and state security systems. As a knowledge elite, they will also play a vital role in shaping how society responds to challenges such as scientific revolutions in genetics and nanotechnology, as well as increasing divisions between rich and poor and environmental degradation.

- The privatisation of global health care may be tamed towards coherence with foundational social and professional virtues through a greater worldwide institutional emphasis on policing, administering and financing global public goods. This will assist work towards an acceptable vision for the sustainable (over millions of years) existence of humans on Earth.

Case study: Ngaire's story

In Peru, diarrhoea kills more than 7000 children annually; it is Peru's second biggest killer of children under 5. In this context, the successful clinical trial of an anti-diarrheal drug manufactured by a US biotechnology company (derived from rice genetically engineered to produce two key proteins, lactoferrin and lysozyme, in mother's milk) should have been acclaimed as a revolutionary breakthrough for global public health. Yet US rice farmers feared genetically engineered rice would inadvertently mix with their crops and limit their marketing. Their political influence resulted in no such 'biopharmed' drug achieving quality and safety market approval from the global benchmark US FDA. What guidance should an 'integrated' system of medical professional regulation give to Ngaire, a doctor working in Peru, about this problem?

Case study: Lucy's story

A doctor was approached by the parents of a teenage girl of normal weight who had gone out to purchase an over-the-counter weight loss drug after seeing an advertisement for it on TV. The pharmaceutical's manufacturer had recently broadcast a television commercial for an anti-obesity drug during episodes of *Idol*, a TV program popular amongst teenagers. Such an advertisement was in breach of therapeutic goods regulations against unnecessary advertising or advertising for clinical indications (disease conditions) that had not been approved by that regulator. The National Drugs and Poisons Scheduling Committee (NDPSC) had given final permission for consumer advertising of the new weight loss drug only a few months earlier, after a campaign lasting 18 months, having recently rescheduled the product from prescription to 'pharmacist-only'. Under an 'integrated' system of professional regulation, should health professionals, medicines safety regulators and policy-makers accept industry self-regulation in such an instance, or does protecting public health demand more significant fines and penalties?

8

**MEDICAL
PROFESSIONALISM
IN
AN
IDEAL
GLOBAL
SOCIETY**

I. Reconceptualising medicine's social contract in the age of corporate globalisation

§i. Recreating universal health care under a new global social contract

Imagine that some time in the future (perhaps after a devastating social crisis), governments are elected in influential developed nations with a mandate to recreate systems of universal (taxpayer-funded and egalitarian) health care.

The public in those nations may have had fond memories of the period when if any person suffered the misfortune of severe accidental injury, they would be cared for, without charge and regardless of private health insurance status, by a public hospital system that equitably provided high quality of care. Many could also recall the systems through which cost-effectiveness experts bargained down, and their government reimbursed from taxation revenue, most of the price of prescription pharmaceuticals. Not a few may have become dissatisfied with being asked to view themselves as consumers (voiceless except as shareholders), rather than citizen owners, of the health care system.

The new governments pass legislation and allocate appropriate monies to establish a system of public hospitals. Such hospitals are to be located on compulsorily acquired prime real estate overlooking beaches or lakes, or with views of distant mountains. Medical schools are funded to construct buildings nearby, to facilitate clinical training. Under new health policies, carers of the aged, the disabled or the chronically ill receive 'social credit' points, which become an implicit currency redeemable as, for example, reduced public transportation or medication co-payment costs.

Nations likewise now can earn credits against their foreign debt and trade imbalances (on a global reserve currency system) by being certified as upholding specified international human rights and global public goods. Examples of ways to earn such public goods policy credits include reducing pollution, assisting biodiversity, protecting the common cultural and natural heritage of humanity, punishing corruption, setting up carbon sequestration schemes, using renewable energy, and contributing to peace and demilitarisation.

Medical and pharmaceutical research and development will now be linked to global health priorities through a coordinated treaty-based UN funding and review system. Under the same treaty, safety, quality, efficacy and cost-effectiveness analysis of new health technologies is to be performed by collaborating assessment agencies in different countries, and funded independently of industry, by a tax on global financial transactions (penalising short-horizon round trips, while negligibly affecting incentives for commodity trade or long-term capital investments). Nations are required to measure economic performance against the United Nations' Human Development Index (HDI) rather than using Gross National Product (GNP), which is only a measure of marketed production.

Multinational corporations are now required to be licensed by a UN organisation. The conditions of such charters – themselves regularly reviewed – mandate goals involving both increasing shareholder profits and fulfilling negotiated service requirements concerning the welfare of a specific community and of humanity generally. Such corporations must also pay a specific tax (not applicable to individual humans) each time their equipment and employees use (and thereby degrade) a public good such as airspace (through carbon emissions), oceans (by risk of oil pollution), roads (by risk of collision and surface erosion), the stock exchange (established by taxpayer funds), the legal system (burdening scarce court time), and public-funded universities or regulatory organisations. Fines are imposed on such private organisations for collusion, corruption, workplace human rights abuses or unauthorised influence on democratic processes, including elections. These new governments ask health professionals (a concept now widely recognised as including health corporation executives and policy-makers) for leadership in promoting such policies.

Instead, some multinational corporations use their control over the mass media to portray these changes as undermining global financial stability. They lobby politicians and government officials, arguing that such policies should again be contrary to WTO rules – which once required massive compensation payouts to adversely affected corporations. They ensure that academics at institutes they fund produce learned articles and opinion-editorial pieces highlighting the problems of such reforms, including that they undermine economic growth, erode quality health care, hamper the production of life-saving new therapies, reduce staff motivation and eliminate incentives for managers to do more good than the legislated standards require them to do. They appeal to health professionals to support their campaign against such reforms.

A useful analogy as to how coherence reasoning within an 'integrated' system of professional regulation could assist resolution of such a dilemma in a post-market state world may be found in Hermann Hesse's Nobel Prize-winning novel *The Glass Bead Game*. The title refers to an eclectic 'game' played by the monastic spiritual guardians of future nation states. Players of the Glass Bead Game, just like leaders of modern medical professionalism, must become adept at achieving coherence amongst principles from areas of learning as diverse as music, history, philosophy, art, architecture, literature, mathematics, anatomy, physiology, pathology, pharmacology, mystical theology, moral philosophy, bioethics, health law and international human rights.[1]

Such a coherence process of professional reasoning is infinitely more complex than simply relying on the limited range of principles derived from either positive law or market fundamentalism. It is, however, likely to gain considerable legitimacy, long term, from inter-generational community approval of its encouragement of conscience and virtue. This chapter presents some concluding reflections on its components, strengths and weaknesses as part of a professional regulatory system moving beyond the age of the market state.

§ii. Human rights and 'integrated' professional regulation in a new global social contract

An evidence-based approach to redefining the foundational features of a regulatory system for health professionals in the post-market state era might have involved determining and analysing a statistically significant number of relatively uncontroversial typical instances. The purpose would not have been to provide a complete set of necessary and sufficient conditions. Rather, it would have been to highlight characteristics most easily recognised and supported by a relevant population sample. Such a method, to be valid, however, would have required extensive and sophisticated sociological research and the resultant data would undoubtedly be subject to a large number of distorting and confounding variables.

This work has turned instead to the well-established intellectual notion of a hypothetical social contract seeking to establish and sustain that increasingly controversial entity known as a just, peaceful, democratic society. It has posited the important role – in creating principles and rules – not only of great social virtues (such as justice and respect for human dignity), but also of a coordinating professional virtue (loyalty to the relief of patient suffering). It has also highlighted the fact that corporations, being artificial persons, inherently lack those natural biological drives that support families or communities, or develop virtues. This is so regardless of the extent to which laws or sound executive leadership may push them in that direction. This text has sought to suggest ways in which corporations may be systematically factored into such idealistic deliberations, to the advantage of social and professional policy.

Some scholars, as we have seen, consider rights to be fundamental to the regulation of any ideal social or professional arrangement, to balance self-interested calculations inimical to duty. This emphasis on legal rights appears to imply a combination of both self-assurance about their universal regulatory importance and mistrust of fellow citizens to uphold them. At the conceptual heart of any workable social contract, such theorists contend, must be the presumption of mutual promises, contractual-type guarantees involving rules about when any one person's freedom can be interfered with by another, and statements about the aims of the collective. Yet competitive individualism of the type valorised by free market theorists sees a need for enforceable legal rights, chiefly to prevent crime and promote national security, or for when important individual human or corporate objectives cannot be achieved by generally acceptable business tactics.

The drafters of the *Universal Declaration of Human Rights* saw international human rights as inherent in the ideal social contract for global civil society they were trying to create. Foundational ethical principles derived from, say, professional virtues such as loyalty to the relief of patient suffering are readily conceived as coherent with human rights principles requiring respect for bodily integrity, inherent dignity and sanctity of life. The theorists of market fundamentalism and corporate globalisation have rarely attempted to achieve such conceptual coherence, except in an apparently tokenistic way (the monetarist position that liberty equals corporate freedom to exploit the market, for example). This lack of explicit engagement with the great ideals of humanity has threatened a catastrophic loss of democratic legitimacy for, and citizen disengagement from, market state institutions and ideology which no amount of public relations 'spin' has been able to rectify.

In the post-market state era, international human rights will still have to overcome suspicions that they are cultural products of a Western liberal political tradition. Those who support them will have to answer claims that these rights do not satisfy the legal positivist sources thesis, or secondary rules of recognition, and so if added, for example, to international trade agreements, would allow an element of unacceptable uncertainty and unpredictability to adjudication. The legitimacy of such assertions, however, is undermined by the inclusion of non-violation nullification of benefits (NVNB) clauses in trade agreements during the market state era. NVNB rules allow threats of trade sanctions against nations for breaching only the 'spirit' of deliberately vague (constructively ambiguous) provisions (such as respect for 'innovation' in medicines policy).

Beyond the age of the market state, increasingly powerful enforcement mechanisms for international law, plus constitutional, legislative and common law requirements on judges to routinely use such norms in adjudication, will see international human rights playing an increasingly important role in health professional regulation.

§iii. *Health technology regulation in a new global social contract*

One of the big tasks of medical professionalism, as the era of the market state draws to a close, may be to play a role in the establishment of a global regulatory architecture that expresses a much better balance between private and public goods in the development and use of health technologies.

Such global health policy proposals will represent a different emphasis from those that encouraged wealthy states and philanthropic foundations to give poor nations greater consumer buying power to attract pharmaceutical research and development for neglected diseases. Examples of the latter approach included the Advance Market Commitment vaccination scheme. This involved guaranteed purchase of a specified number of treatments, at a pre-set price, of vaccines against rotavirus, pneumococcal disease, human papilloma virus, malaria, HIV/AIDS and tuberculosis. Sponsors would pay only when research had confirmed a new drug's quality, safety, efficacy and cost-effectiveness, as would the poorest countries, whose contribution would be a low co-payment for each dose.

Similarly, the Clinton Foundation used pooled resources from France, Brazil, Britain, Norway and Chile (raised from taxes on airline tickets) to bargain discounts on 3-in-1 anti-HIV/AIDS drugs from Indian manufacturers Cipla and Ranbaxy. This allowed the treatment of over 100,000 children in 40 nations in 2007 at a cost of approximately US$60 per person a year. Such systems, though making valuable contributions, left untouched the inequities implicit in the continued dominance of private profit-focused rights in global health technology research and development.

Equally friendly to multinational corporate interests have been suggestions that self-governance, corporate responsibility and corporate philanthropy should be allowed to remedy the problem, through compassionate use schemes, public–private partnerships, or manufacturer contributions to charities that offer its drug at discount prices.

The post-market state era may see the practical realisation of more visionary and public goods-focused approaches to global health technology research and development. One such strategy has been developed by Jamie Love and staff at CP-Tech, with the assistance of numerous eminent academics and health policy-makers. It involves replacing intellectual property (patent) marketing monopolies for all prescription drugs with 'prize fund' payments (0.5 per cent of GDP) rewarding inventions proven to improve health care outcomes, as measured by Quality Adjusted Life Years (QALYs) or other metrics now used by governments and insurance companies.

Such efforts led to a 2006 resolution of the World Health Assembly (the policy-making body of the WHO). This committed the WHO to investigate blueprinting a new system of prioritising and financing pharmaceutical research aimed at stimulating the development of drugs, vaccines and diagnostics for diseases that member states identify as health priorities.[2] One of the most important suggestions in the resolution was that incentives for research and development should be linked to health outcomes. In December 2006, the five-day WHO Intergovernmental Working Group (IGWG) meeting on public health, innovation and intellectual property, involving representatives from many important NGOs, as well as states, showed itself to be another important vehicle through which the elements of such a new global social contract on health technology development might arise.

A related global public goods initiative could involve negotiations towards a specific UN or WHO *Treaty on Universal Health Care*. This would establish norms requiring benchmark targets of health service delivery and improvements in health care areas such as those listed in the United Nations' Millennium Development Goals (for example). Such an instrument would obligate states to accept that schemes for taxpayer-funded universal health care, like the human genome, or natural and cultural places of significance, represent part of the common heritage of humanity.

Synergistic with (or perhaps incorporated within) the above initiatives could be a multilateral *Treaty on Safety and Cost-Effectiveness Assessment of Health Technologies*. This treaty would appropriately and sustainably reward medicines and medical device 'innovation', after internationally harmonised expert pre-marketing assessment of the scientific evidence for its safety, quality, efficacy, and cost-effectiveness. Such assessments, funded by a tax on global financial transactions, would build upon the effectiveness of the WHO essential medicines list.

This treaty would create mechanisms whereby global civil society could work towards principles for clinical trial design that are more responsive to the global burden of disease. Treaty working parties and committees would negotiate to establish the general principles and detailed mechanisms for globally orchestrated parallel and shared evaluations, both pre-marketing and post-marketing. It would similarly coordinate global conditional approvals based on binding outcome agreements, consistent and transparent assessment of linked usage and outcome data, best use of surrogate outcomes or modelling, increased disclosure of marginal cost of production, and better governance of industry commercial-in-confidence claims over clinical trial data (transparent, protective of public safety, and not made unilaterally). The treaty and its funding would also cover liability protection and indemnity for assessors.

Such a treaty would have the advantage of not interfering with existing patent protection standards for medicines and medical devices. It would not become a barrier to market access for innovative products. It would rather attempt to ensure that the prices nations paid for such new medical technologies, through reimbursement schemes, represented clinical value when compared with already marketed therapeutic goods.

One of the main tasks of the committees established under this treaty would be to work towards a more rational approach to price-setting for new, allegedly innovative, patented medicines and medical devices. Independent regulatory officials representing the global community interest will be better able to assess such prices (even on a commercial-in-confidence basis) against progressively more accurate and objective data on marginal cost of production. Other issues could involve working towards linkage of every clinical use of a new health technology with health outcome data from an individual (de-identified) medical record. Such a treaty would enhance public trust in regulators, so removing one of the main causes of share price volatility and capital flights. It would also facilitate sustainable returns for industry.

§iv. *Professional conscience and natural law in a new global social contract*

The 'integrated' professional regulatory system proposed here is designed to stimulate development of conscience and character (or virtue). Many legal scholars and policy-makers, as mentioned, may view such features as incompatible with consistent and predictable application of rules and rights, and as involving a reformulated 'natural law' position. Yet beyond the age of the market state, scientific research may make stronger claims for the practical existence of conscience and of natural law principles derived from the study of human interactions and psychology.

Natural law is closely related to the idea of principles and rules arising from a social contract concerning individual liberties and distribution of public goods. Both were previously often caricatured as a type of arch nemesis of legal positivism, much as virtue ethics was frequently considered the intellectual opposite of an ethics of principles and duty. Yet history confirms the claims of pure reason: that the more the content and processes of governance systems withdraw support from foundational social virtues, such as justice and respect for human dignity, the greater their chance of being considered illegitimate and thus being short-lived. Public relations 'spin' and advertising, or repression of dissidents, can delay, but not prevent, the consequent decline of these governance systems.

One relevant natural law idea (also called the Radbruch Thesis), as previously mentioned, holds that a fundamentally (or 'intolerably') unjust statute should not in fact be considered a law by citizens of good conscience. The explanation is that such a moral travesty of law violates those social virtues and derived universally applicable principles (many now incorporated in the corpus of international human rights) that most people's reason (but obviously not always the majority's) tells them ought to be upheld in any society supporting the notion of a basic social contract between citizens and government.

This type of virtue and conscience-related natural law theory emphasises a type of coherence reasoning similar to that posited here as applying within an 'integrated' professional regulatory system. It should be distinguished from the caricature version which the legal scholar Hans Kelsen criticised as paving the way for the infamous totalitarian regimes of the mid-20th century. Kelsen disliked natural law because he believed that it jurisprudentially grounded the authority of the state in intolerant mystico-religious ideologies lacking a basis in anthropological fact, rather than on rule by more objective processes of law.[3] Kelsen's main concern was to prevent natural law conceptually justifying absolute state power over its citizens.

Health corporation executives and policy-makers implementing the ideology of market fundamentalism are likely to view themselves as 'neutralists', who believe that laws should simply provide a minimally efficient framework within which each consumer can pursue the good, as he or she understands it (often under the influence of the mass media). Neutralism draws support from communities in which the leadership is not willing to promote informed rigorous public debate about fundamental values and ways of living, and is instead prepared to hand over governance in key areas of society to managers and alleged experts. A version of this approach is known, in classical rhetoric, as an *argumentum ad verecundiam*, an argument that demands acceptance merely out of deference to the prestige, stature and presumed authority of the person, institution or office propounding it.

'Integrated' professional regulation, on the other hand, seeks a coherence between a natural law emphasis on individual conscience and a positive law promotion of predictability and consistency in legal process. Once practical regulatory systems and institutions begin to actively promote conscience in this way, that will become a socially powerful ideal. It will encourage resistance to values and processes that oppose the development of foundational social and professional virtues through consistent application of universally applicable principles as expressed in, for example, bioethics and international human rights.

Also strongly emphasising a link between legalism and natural law, between the rule of law and questions of virtue and conscience, are theorists termed 'governmentalists', or 'perfectionists'. Health professionals (including health corporation executives and policy-makers) supporting this position are likely to acknowledge that good laws play a major role in whether or not citizens aspire to become virtuous, capable of preferring the public good to their own selfish interests, able to consistently apply universally applicable principles despite protracted opposition.

Such 'normative' (or principle and rule-creating) idealism, as we have seen, has a venerable pedigree in Western civilisation.[4] Far from being merely emotivist (a strange but common form of conceptual deprecation amongst particular types of intellectuals), the enduring value of an idealistic approach to norm creation may be seen in the historical transformation of natural law ideals into laws. Such ideals (about human emancipation, dignity and self-realisation free from state interference, for example), as discussed, moved from the conscience, virtue and reason of theorists such as Locke and Thomas Paine into general social consciousness, and then found imperfect expression in foundational legal documents such as the *Virginia Declaration of Rights 1776*, the *American Declaration of Independence 1776*, the French *Déclaration des Droits de l'Homme et du Citoyen 1789* and ultimately the United Nations' *Universal Declaration on Human Rights* of 1948, particularly Article 1:[5]

All beings are born free and equal in dignity and rights.
They are endowed with reason and conscience and should act
towards one another in a spirit of brotherhood.

It has already been mentioned that a powerful measure of the social
legitimacy of health professionals and their system of regulation
will be how they treat whistleblowers. Popular opinion will judge
both industry and the profession generally harshly for excessively
marginalising such courageous and principled professionals by,
for example, bringing or threatening defamation actions against
them, contractually limiting their free speech as employees and
restricting their freedom of association through workplace legislation.
Communities have probably learnt well during the era of the market
state that it is often only through whistleblowers, motivated by loyalty
to the relief of patient suffering, that they learn of the genuine risks
of health care institutions and new technologies.

This being so, it will be a duty of medical professionalism, as the
world emerges from the age of the market state, to treat whistleblowing
seriously and integrate it into clinical governance pathways. This is
more likely to occur if health care whistleblowing has an established
conceptual base in academic theory, as an inheritor not only of
natural law, but also of civil disobedience law reform and virtue
ethics traditions.[6] Similarly important will be its respect in policy-
making processes, and in legislation offering protection from reprisals
and possibly *qui tam* payments of a proportion of the public monies
recovered, if the allegation is proven.

§v. Medical professionalism and social leadership beyond the age of the market state

Why should a doctor or health policy-maker be well placed to offer
social as well as professional leadership for the public good beyond the
age which promoted a fully privatised global health care system?

Health professionals (whether clinicians, managers, corporate
executives or policy-makers) will be trained to understand and
communicate the regulatory implications of duties flowing primarily

from a society's collective desire that its citizens exhibit virtues, such as concern for others, justice and equity. Further, their career training under an 'integrated' system of professional regulation will require them to participate in (or observe) intrusions upon patients that are not always directly relevant to relief of those patients' suffering. The knowledge health professionals thereby gain should be regarded as held in trust for the community of future patients, not bargained away as if it were individual property.

Recognition of the primal regulatory importance of communal caring about public health underpins recommendations that professionalism be placed at the core of medicine's social contract.[7] The next generation of health care professionals, however, if they are to become effective patient advocates and social leaders, need to understand and learn from the way the market state once attempted to manipulate the outward symbols and processes of political democracy, and even of traditional medical ethics.

In the age beyond the market state, problem-based learning scenarios, to prepare health professionals for social leadership roles, should include exploring how health technology corporations can facilitate what are now legislated goals: long-term sustainable industry profits for shareholders and availability of health care services and affordable quality medicines. Curricula should modify traditional instruction in medical ethics and health law to instead deal with how such norms can provide leadership criteria for corporate lobbying strategies. Students could learn how to balance moral, ethical, legal and human rights, on the one hand, with, on the other, responsibilities emerging from a new global social contract that reinterprets what were multinational corporate policy lobbying devices (or trade agreement 'constructive ambiguities').

'Transparency' claims, for example, should require a *quid pro quo* between disclosure of regulatory processes and limitation on corporate commercial-in-confidence protections. 'Fast-track' safety, quality, efficacy and cost-effectiveness regulatory approval processes must be accepted as having enforceable public interest limits. 'Recognition of pharmaceutical innovation' similarly should be recognised as involving expert objective demonstration of both a new product's therapeutic significance and its value in a market appropriately regulated to ensure genuine competition. 'Liberalisation of trade in hospital services' likewise should be redefined by a normatively more 'integrated' WTO to allow re-establishment of taxpayer-funded egalitarian health care schemes as a natural (and non-compensable) part of a market required to genuinely respect 'freedom' in terms of both individual human rights and the rights of societies to democratically mandate non-profit approaches to service provision. Any industry demand to remove or 'dismantle discriminatory price controls' should be supervised by global anti-monopoly regulators that seek to ensure a policy balance between the aims of multinational corporations and of central government health technology cost-effectiveness expert evaluation systems.

II. Critical reflections on the ideal approach

§i. *Idealistic collective policy goals may threaten individual liberties*

Apologists for the market state might dismiss the type of idealistic approach to medical professionalism and leadership proposed here as merely a harmless academic pastime. They could claim that it, like other medical professionalism renewal projects, appears to lack any reasonable prospect of making economically or politically useful global policy change. How is it possible, their argument might run, for health corporation executives and government health policy-makers to see any financial advantage in actively promoting governance systems founded on vague universal ideals and related professional or social virtues, bioethical principles, laws or international human rights? Why shouldn't clinical medicine be promoted as simply about repairing dysfunction in progressively more wealthy 'consumers' with freedom of choice?

Such critics might further argue that there is only a difference in degree between founding regulation of medical professionalism on social and professional virtues, on the one hand, and plans to assist all human societies to coalesce on the governance model of a mass media-influenced, nominally democratic free-market state, on the other. Both approaches appear, they could claim, only truly compatible with societies whose citizens have homogenous goals.

John Rawls, for instance, in developing his influential conception of legal principles as evolving from social contract respect for the foundational social virtue of justice, opposed 'perfectionist' governance positions where the state attempts to enforce its vision of a collective form of *eudaimonia*. He claimed that such policies readily make individual liberties subservient to transient political or religious ideologies (such as socialism, economic rationalism, neoconservatism, communism, right-wing Christianity or Islam), instead of firmly rooting them in universally applicable principles.[8] The eugenics movement in 1930s (so dangerously misinterpreted and overlooked by Flexner's recommendations for reform of medical education) could be regarded as but one salutary example in the health care context. More contemporary instances are the mass murders perpetrated by Pol Pot's regime in Cambodia and the 'ethnic cleansing' implemented in the former Yugoslavia.

Universal regulatory ideals, it may further be objected, are the uncertain products of contentious idealist philosophical schools (such as the Grand Theory tradition, Enlightenment, or International Civil Society projects). This tends to limit endorsement of their related principles in practical contemporary policy debates. A foundational principle of medical professionalism such as respect for patient autonomy, for instance, could be described as merely a preferred instrument for achieving a liberal-individualist culture. Reason, the primary tool used to construct such ideal principles, may itself actually have been moulded by association with historical governance systems aiming primarily at the satisfaction of vices such as greed through social power and dominance. A regulatory system's focus on specific social and professional virtues arguably provides a contentious and even divisive normative baseline in a pluralist society.

Further, some scholars might contend that there is no particular reason for, or evidence about, why such a high degree of normative coherence should be sought in a professional regulatory system. Indeed, the achievement of justice in a democratic community, they might maintain, could well require that the law not be judicially interpreted as speaking with one voice. Occasional acts that are incoherent with domestic legal regimes may be necessary, particularly in 'failed' states or dysfunctional societies, to advance human rights protections.

Coherence theories resembling that proposed here could also be conceptually attacked as placing the primary sources of critique inside the law-making system, thus marginalising the lobbying role of NGOs and grass-roots community non-violent protest and civil disobedience in promoting the international human rights agenda. Further, judges, legislators and health policy-makers under common law and civil code systems are likely to frame issues, reason and use legal principles about medical professionalism in different ways. There is a divergence in substance and not just form, it thus could be claimed, between the French *Conseil d'Etat*'s or *Cour de cassation*'s application of public order (*l'ordre public*) or good morals (*bonnes moeurs*) and the German *Bundesverfassungsgericht*'s use of appropriateness (*geeignet*) and necessity (*erforderlich*) with respect to legislation, that no amount of appealing to 'coherence' reasoning will overcome.[9]

Yet encouraging health professionals (including health corporation executives and policy-makers) to view themselves as part of an international 'community of principle' should make them more receptive to, for example, the calibrating roles of both extra-jurisdictional bioethics and international human rights. This should make it less likely that any particular decision made under an 'integrated' system of medical professional regulation will narrow upon a conclusive single voice and require the stifling of criticism.

Similarly, foundational virtues actually provide the least contentious sources for derivation of regulatory principle. They appear to be an inescapable component of moral psychology. Even in the most oppressive circumstances, such as in concentration camps, in gulags and under torture, intuitive convictions and emotions about foundational virtues are the last part of humanity to perish. Compassion towards human suffering is an inescapable regulatory fact in health care institutions. Any governance arrangements in this area will benefit from genuinely acknowledging and prioritising it in institutional governance structures.

Making the role of conscience in enunciation of legal norms more explicit and transparent strengthens the legitimacy of both professional regulation and state and corporate governance. It makes it less likely that a community will disengage from its judiciary, legislative process, or even health care system, because they appear to be dominated by uninspiring profit-making interests.

§ii. *Vulnerability of a single fountain or spring*

Vincent van Gogh's letters describe the artist using colour in portraits as a means of depicting character. He mentions painting his friend Dr Gachet, for example, in a glorious profusion of 'virtues' which appear to reflect Vincent's empathy for suffering undergone, both physically and in affairs of the heart, while staying true to the higher spiritual aims of a practice, be it medicine or art.[10]

The doctor or health policy-maker who consistently performs the moral duties created by his or her 'internalisation' of professional norms may indeed be described as possessing many virtues. Fidelity to promises and obligations, veracity and empathy, for example, are frequently referred to in this context. So are compassion and empathy focused directly on another's good. Also present are more self-regarding virtues such as sagacity, circumspection, and Osler's *aequanimitas*, which involves a greater emphasis on principled action. Finally, there are 'mixed' virtues such as courage.

One problem with the use of such a list of virtues in a functional regulatory strategy such as this is that, as we have seen, it can never be definitive or permanent. For a variety of cultural and historical reasons, the requirements of such virtues may conflict, either generally or in different clinical circumstances. Such a list would inevitably lead to unnecessary and unproductive academic and professional comparisons between virtues. It would become controversial and clumsy in educational settings. It may lack the inspirational focus that comes from habitually linking intuitive convictions, emotion and fundamental principle in a regulatory context with a single, clear ideal.

The foundational and unifying professional virtue of loyalty to the relief of patient suffering, as the single 'fountain' or 'spring' of professional regulatory principle, may be subject to the previously discussed criticisms of 'coherence' theories of jurisprudence. Perhaps it is wrong, for example, for such a theory to posit that proximity to individual patient suffering either directly, or indirectly through the medical humanities, inevitably arouses professional conscience.

Some people like to look at images of acute suffering, delight in the pains and misfortunes of others and eagerly pursue the spectacle of a grievous calamity, the love of cruelty seeming as natural to them as sympathy.[11] But is this true of all human beings, regardless of their education? Does it apply, for example, to those professionals who have been taught to value virtue, to train their conscience and respect the traditions that encourage its allegiance to ideals of human welfare? It could be argued that there are in all parts of society people who enjoy things you and I think of as immoral, to say the least. Can training of any kind truly affect these things?

Further, an 'integrated' system of regulation based on such a professional virtue might appear to have a circular logic: the virtuous health professional or policy-maker is one who seeks virtue (either in him or herself, or in their immediate organisation or community). Let loose in a professional regulatory system, this unstable concept, allegedly promoting a fragile, loosely defined cosmopolitanism, could interfere with certainty and predictability in the application of legal rules. It could undermine their power to challenge, for example, patterns of structural bias that favour managerial sovereignty by knowledge elites.

A regulatory emphasis on loyalty to the relief of patient suffering may similarly be considered simply to endorse unstructured, intuitive cognition. Involving conscience so directly, and allowing bioethics and international human rights to become calibration systems for law, may only lead to incessant controversy about not only the content of law, but what 'law' is. This could promote an ineffective regulatory oscillation – between despondent apologies for manifest failures and bursts of optimistic utopian policy – whose apparent cumulative ineffectiveness gradually undermines the confidence of regulatory idealists and pushes them into petty struggles for legitimisation by the state.

Finally, a regulatory emphasis on loyalty to the relief of patient suffering could be objected to as encouraging unpredictable, potentially chaotic and even dangerous acts of conscientious non-compliance or civil disobedience when legal rules are determined by doctors not to fit coherently with related ethical and human rights principles. Conscience, redolent with notions of intuition and emotion, may thus be seen as an inadequate basis for efficient decision-making in modern, high-tech societies. A health professional's excessive reliance on conscience in such deliberations, such an argument might continue, harkens back to the age when medicine was a priestly function.

I argue, though, that no amount of mass media consumerist indoctrination, promotion of debt and financial insecurity, and reduction of time and capacity for community participation will ever permanently induce the majority of citizens and health professionals to renounce conscience or their commitment to social and professional virtues. The urge to remedy (rather than financially exploit) another's suffering will remain a crucial distinguishing feature of health care systems. Only governance and regulatory structures which manifestly support this truth will prosper in the long term.

§iii. More power as capricious consumers and shareholders?

Simone de Beauvoir wrote *A Very Easy Death* about her mother's hospitalisation during terminal illness. It is a memoir that vividly describes the variety of tensions and power imbalances likely to remain implicit in the health care transaction:

> Would Dr P keep his promise: 'She shall not suffer'? A race
> had begun between death and [medical treatment in the guise
> of] torture. I asked myself how one manages to go on living
> when someone you love has called out to you 'Have pity on
> me' in vain. And even if death were to win, all this odious
> deception! Maman thought that we were with her, next to
> her; but we were already placing ourselves on the far side of

her history. An evil all-knowing spirit, I could see behind
the scenes, while she was struggling, far, far away, in human
loneliness. Her desperate eagerness to get well, her patience,
her courage – it was all deceived. She would not be paid for any
of her sufferings at all. I saw her face again: 'Since it is good for
me.'[12]

In a fully privatised global health care system, the primary *telos* or
goal of medical professionalism might have been argued (by business
managers and health policy-makers) to most profitably and efficiently
involve helping only consumers who can readily be perceived as 'good'.
Relevant examples of 'good' in this context might have included
consumers making useful choices about their wellbeing and building
up their health savings accounts, or being willing to prioritise the
cost of quality health care in their lives. More contentiously, it could
also have involved those wealthy enough to support the system by
taking out adequate private health insurance, or becoming investors
or shareholders in health care corporations. Such interpretations are
extensions of the view that direct responsibility for structural changes
in global health care should best rest with a deregulated marketplace.

These ideas, however, consign many of the world's poor, aged and
disabled to the second-class status of being recipients of 'safety net'
care. This health policy expression, perhaps unwittingly, captures
both a subtle denigration of such people as unable to perform on the
corporate high wire and the sub-standard medicine they are likely
to fall upon. It denies the relevance to health policy or medical
professionalism of according all patients a respect for their inherent
human dignity. Further, research data showing that the market actions
of most consumers and stockholders are generally capricious tends to
nullify arguments that free markets can, in the absence of effective
state regulation, effectively distribute scarce resources in health care.

Health alone, it has been argued here, cannot be the primary good
or *telos* of medical professionalism. Many would object to this, saying
that doctors should be primarily urged to be less disease-focused, more
concerned with preventive medicine, with health impact assessments
of policy, with the whole person, with physical, mental and social
wellbeing. Some might even claim that a logical extension of such

ideas is that health policy-makers should be more open to promoting health and medicines savings accounts, or managed care plans (either taxpayer or private health insurance funded) that focus on prophylactic measures aimed at circumventing hospitalisations.

But the existence of health (rather than suffering), as has been said above, cannot be presumed to immediately arouse the conscience of a health professional (including a health corporation executive or policy-maker) to implement universally applicable principles with any deep-rooted emotive urgency. A system of medical professionalism that is not fundamentally predicated on the unique fact of individual patients' vulnerability or suffering could lead to a disempowering of the ill, by severing them from traditional normative protections.

Further, we have seen that medicine is made up of many practices that have 'internal' (or primarily personally relevant) goods, such as pleasure in skilful surgical technique, perspicacious diagnosis, compassionate presence and esteem as a good teacher. Health professionals (broadly conceived) are privileged in their career. Financially exploited workers in clothing industry sweatshops, forced prostitutes, conscripted child soldiers, people struggling to provide enough shelter, food and water for their families, for example, are not in the fortunate position of being able to view their career as a process of character development rather than a struggle for survival.

The need to balance this medical privilege with responsibility is another factor that supports action for the relief of individual patient suffering, rather than achievement of patient 'good', as the primary goal of an 'integrated' regulatory system for medical professionalism. Such a goal is designed to operate in much the same way as the influential legal scholar Edmond Cahn's concept of 'injustice' does in the context of law reform.

The relevant assumptions, in each case, are twofold. First, that conscience is most likely to be aroused by proximity to individual human vulnerability and suffering.[13] Second, that conscience so stimulated should be recognised by privatised systems seeking socially valuable action as providing the motive force for consistent patient care in sustainably profitable markets.

§iv. Is medical professionalism and leadership inherently elitist and paternalistic?

Tolstoy's *Death of Ivan Ilyich* depicts a magistrate who has perfected in his daily work a technique of 'eliminating all considerations irrelevant to the legal aspect of the case'. Now, in his final illness, 'the airs that he put on in court for the benefit of the prisoner at the bar, the doctor now put on for him'.

Tolstoy contrasts the friendly, loyal servant Gerassim, who becomes Ilyich's nurse, with the haughty, condescending, prevaricating, but celebrated medical specialist. He describes the unpretentious and honest way in which the former cleans, positions and comforts the patient, who otherwise feels that 'he and his pain were being thrust somewhere into a narrow, deep, black sack'. Even more insight can be gained from such passages if it is recalled that one of the chief iconoclasts and critics of medical professionalism in the 20th century wrote under the name of Ivan Illich.[14]

Doctors, like all professionals, also have to balance subjectively important 'internal' goods connected with their family, relatives and friends, their colleagues and institution, alongside professional duty to their patients. This is an aspect of what Aristotle termed *phronesis* and Thomas Aquinas termed *prudentia*: practical wisdom.

A major objection to the role of professional virtues and related principles in this 'integrated' regulatory system might be that they promote a tendency for doctors and health policy-makers to become self-centred egoists. Surely, these critics argue, this was the problem with the guild or gentleman's club mentality, which focused primarily on issues of etiquette and devalued patients' inherent right to dignity.

The distinction between a desire to achieve goods *internal* to the practice of medicine (character development) and a desire to achieve goods flowing from it *externally* (money, prestige) can indeed devolve into a pantomime show of the former in order to gain the latter. Tolstoy makes this point symbolically in the *Death of Ivan Ilyich* by having the wife of the dying magistrate hand the celebrated specialist his fee with tears in her eyes, just after that physician has disturbed the patient with false hopes of recovery.

This objection also suggests that fully operationalising an 'integrated' regulatory system might lead to worse outcomes for patients, in that self-centred or incompetent doctors might obtain unwarranted advantages from appearing to practise with consistent care and consideration. Further, a regulatory emphasis on a doctor's professional virtue could be viewed as making the acquisition of such character traits dependent on accumulated positive patient outcomes, and thus to some extent on chance, or what is termed moral luck.

Also, in practice, almost all health professionals, at least periodically, will become focused on their own life narrative. Loyalty to the relief of patient suffering then becomes a second-string priority, behind concern about family or preferment, for example. Pressure to obtain research grants, professorial appointments, departmental seniority, or some other form of kudos are all accepted parts of career development that readily accentuate egotistic negative traits and leave health professionals less likely to develop the respect and consideration for another person that lies at the heart of character development.

A related objection would be that such a virtue-based system of regulation, with its insider perspective, merely perpetuates the power of this professional elite to socially marginalise some categories of patients by defining nodal concepts to which ethical and legal duties attach ('disease', 'infertility', 'viability', 'futility' and 'competence', for instance).

A preliminary answer to this 'power elite perpetuation' objection would be that getting more doctors to strive for good character is likely to actually maximise general utility and human rights protection for patients. The chief reason is that it helps to develop an institutional ethos around the consistent performance of duty interpreted according to a broad range of moral, ethical, legal and human rights traditions.

The chief answer to the objection that 'integrated' professional regulation is elitist, however, lies in the other-regarding quality of the foundational professional virtue of loyalty to the relief of patient suffering. It is a recognised paradox (sometimes painfully acquired in idealistic youth) that virtue recedes before egotistic striving for such a worthwhile goal. This highlights the importance in this context of both a practical, socially useful task and what many perceive to be the mysterious role of grace in the pursuit of personal truth. My belief is that in the age beyond the market state, the path to contentment will be widely recognised as involving conscience-directed work.

Loyalty, by definition, arises in the context of relationships. In the post-market state era, any functional regulatory system for health professionals (including health corporation executives and policy-makers) must consider other-regarding virtue because of specific features of the renegotiated global social contract – the nature of illness, and the patient's presumed suffering, vulnerability and need to trust, for example.

Other-regarding virtue is also a required regulatory focus because medical knowledge is not wholly proprietary, but is acquired at a significant financial and personal cost to the community (including, for example, invasion of patient privacy in training). Reinforcing this is the professional oath or public promise to serve the patient and humanity.

It could be argued that emphasising trust and friendship as the key internal regulatory dynamics in medical professionalism would create less risk of implicit power inequality and professional egoism. Yet friendship seems an archaic, unpredictably idiosyncratic and easily manipulated regulatory foundation for a global community emerging from an era of relationship-poor or 'stranger' medicine and shareholder/consumer-dominated governance. In addition, making professional duties initially dependent on proof of a response, such as trust or friendship, would prejudice patients or health professionals with poor communication skills, or patients in whom social disfavour or oppression had produced suspicion or resentment. A regulatory emphasis on friendship might also promote a recrudescence of 'top-down', totalitarian, enforced socialism, with all the attendant problems of loss of human liberty and creativity.

III. Final reflections

§i. Who will champion health care as a global public good?

In 1890, Chekhov determined to pay off some of his 'debt to medicine' by travelling 5000 miles to mountainous Sakhalin Island, Russia's most far-and-forgotten penal settlement, in the wastes of Siberia. Chekhov's sister Marya wrote:

> [A]t that time much was heard of the hard life of the convicts on the island of Sakhalin. People protested and grumbled but that was all. Nobody took any active steps. Anton Pavlovich could not rest after he discovered that convicts suffered so terribly and he decided to go and see for himself.[15]

Chekhov reached Alexandrovsk, the chief town of Sakhalin, on a day when forest fires glowed beyond the mountains and darkened the wharf to but two red lights. Gaining access to data cards, he visited, over the next few months, every man, woman and child on the island. He inspected the prisons. The convicts, he found, slept together in rags and filth: 'It is a beastly existence, it is nihilistic, a negation of proprietary rights, privacy and comfort.'

Why should a regulatory system for medical professionalism beyond the age of the market state place such an emphasis on conscience and the development of virtue? The answer partly lies in the stance this powerful knowledge elite is necessarily required to take in the contest between competing visions of human society.

The age of the market state has been presented here as a theoretical position in which governments are controlled by the will not of the people, but of a particular generation of corporate executives. Such leaders espouse a very limited set of socially and environmentally damaging, profit-driven values. Imbalanced implementation of such values in global health policy risks creating a world where loose gatherings of individualistic consumers grow increasingly apathetic about erosion of their rights and responsibilities as citizens.

Medical professionalism, however, has been forged around the unique foundational regulatory facts of individual patient suffering, vulnerability and need to trust. A case has been made here for institutional support and encouragement of health professionals (including health corporation executives and policy-makers) who seek to achieve virtue through consistently performing actions to relieve such patients' suffering. Their enhanced capacity to do so, despite obstacles, according to principles and rules recognised to have universal application under a renegotiated global social contract, has been presented as likely to strengthen crucial components of the general social fabric.

Any apparent normative circularity (the good is what the good person seeks) is arguably broken here by having this 'integrated' professional regulatory system primarily focused on a unique and independent goal: relieving individual patient suffering. Such regulatory 'integration' is also possible in a health policy sense because commitment in conscience to the construction of any particular virtue readily generates positive principles or rule instructions (just as reflection on a vice spurs a corresponding principle and rule prohibitions). Linkage, in this manner, of virtue theory, principlist ethics and idealist international human rights with the rules of legal positivism brings much of the predictability of the latter to the idealism of the former. It strives to make rule obedience a process of life transformation.

Medical professionalism, so conceived, also carries the promise of enlarging the objects of human sympathy and so the applicable range of principles and rules available to decision-makers.[16] One such principle is 'sustainability', or intergenerational justice. Others are 'cosmopolitanism' (allegiance to global groupings of people committed to universally applicable principles) and 'solidarity' with endangered species and habitats, as well as with the degraded and 'diseased' Earth itself as a self-sustaining organism (the so-called Gaia hypothesis).

The text has gathered together the ingredients for a program which could be an improvement on existing systems of compliance, allocation of responsibility, decision-making in professional regulation and health policy, and education about medical professionalism. Some preliminary testing of its viability and usefulness has been commenced.

Perhaps the most ambitious element of this reconceptualisation of medical professionalism, however, is its attempt to present the relevant careers as modestly efficient methods of character development. It is a regulatory system that attempts to promote a greater symbiosis between conscience, rule obedience and activism for democratic regulatory support of global public goods.

Health professionals under the 'integrated' system of professional regulation presented here are expected to resemble everyday 'heroes', people like author James Joyce's character Bloom, who had an eye of pity and a hand of loyalty amidst trying circumstances. Rather than producing superdoctors who claim to never make errors and earn millions every year from process royalties, shareholdings and perquisites, health professionals under this program are expected to diligently use portable technology to record even 'near-miss' adverse incidents, accept the appropriateness of the patient complaint process and peer review system, be ready to apologise and remain sincerely committed, in corporate governance and health policy debates, to the foundational professional virtue of relief of individual patient suffering.

Possible weaknesses of this 'integrated' approach to regulation of medical professionalism have been explored. They relate chiefly to the challenging demands placed on regulatory participants to lead transparently virtuous lives, to view their careers in terms of conscience and development of character. This may make this 'integrated' approach initially more suitable for use in an educative setting. Another possible frailty is its potential, if wrongly interpreted, to parody corporations as implicitly antisocial, when their desire for sustainable operations may make individual private health care and health technology organisations and CEOs much more responsive over time to the altruistic ideals of humanity.

It must surely be a short-lived era in which the market state succeeds in stripping citizen participation in democracy of genuine impact. The USA, so influential in developing the model of globally privatised health care, undoubtedly will have a vital role to play in helping medical professionalism and society move successfully beyond the age where markets devalued sustainability and conscience.

The age of the market state, with its short-term financial benefits only to the world's wealthy, will probably be looked back upon with a mixture of curiosity and disgust. It will be seen as a time when governments uncritically facilitated a free market ideology that placed a high priority on cutting taxpayer-funded health care services, deregulating, and turning a blind eye to monopoly power, collusion, asymmetries of information and increasing gaps between socio-economic groups in health care access and outcomes. Historians will wonder why global society, in the face of so many substantial threats to collective survival, permitted such corporations for so long to be uncritically supported by taxpayer-funded subsidies, to influence legislation and trade agreements outside normal democratic processes, and to price new health technology products, all without genuine accountability.

As the world emerges from the age of the market state, communities will expect health professionals and policy-makers to perform their career tasks with greater interest in lessening the 'unfreedoms' that lie behind the ostensibly unlimited consumer choices permitted by the market state. Genuine liberty should include the capacity for communities to turn, if they wish, to cosmopolitan identities, intermediate technologies and local sharing of resources – and skills aimed at producing virtues in the process of making goods. WTO rules should be altered to allow societies to return to such universalist models without needing to compensate corporate actors. The championing, by the leaders of medical professionalism, of respect for justice, respect for human dignity, and loyalty to the relief of suffering also may become one of the last great barriers against society's participation in, or tolerance of, atrocity, torture or cruelty.[17]

In this environment, fewer health professionals should need, as a matter of survival, to plan careers in private-owned medicine, large private firms, or government departments dedicated to supporting the needs of private industry. This will make taxpayer support of their education more feasible. No longer under pressure to earn an income during their period of studying, and in a regulatory context in sympathy with global public goods and the great aspirations and ideals of humanity, it will be easier for such students to develop their own conscience and career aspirations.

The market state's self-interested corporate 'brand' loyalty will then be unlikely to effectively replace loyalty to the relief of suffering as the dominant professional motivational factor. That being true, in a thousand years' time (should humanity survive that long) it should still be possible to say that we 'own' our own health.

In the course of many illnesses there comes a point when the patient must accept their own death. All of us reach this point individually. Yet most hang on to the comforting thought that our children and future generations will survive us to continue the human adventure. A turning point in the legitimacy and continued existence of the market state, however, may occur when a majority of people worldwide reach the conclusion that the global suffering produced by free market fundamentalist policies (particularly through their promotion of weapons of mass destruction, poverty, illness, inequality and environmental destruction) has progressed so far that it is, in effect, likely to lead to the death of the entire human species.

Why should we expect the next generation to shoulder the responsibility for rejecting a world where conscience and foundational social and professional virtues have become mere 'brand names', useful mostly in the task of selling health service products?

My conviction is that there is a future for humanity for millions of years beyond the age of the market state, in which there will still be markets and still be states, but the spheres of responsibility for each will be more sensibly and sustainably defined. This time will not be reached by the implementation of any one particular ideology or political program, but by the enhanced capacity of all citizens to make decisions coherent with conscience and with universally applicable principles. An 'integrated' system of medical professionalism will play a crucial leadership role in this process of market 'humanisation'.

Chapter summary and cases for further discussion

- As the era of the market state draws to a close, human society is likely to turn to models of cosmopolitan allegiance (focused on respect for universally applicable principles rather than nationality, culture or narrow religious ideology) and to systems of universal access to health care and health technologies.

- Beyond the age of the market state, a better balance between corporate profits and global public goods in health care can be facilitated by treaties on *Universal Access to Health Care* and *Safety and Cost-Effectiveness Assessment of Health Technologies*, as well as pharmaceutical research and development being better focused on the global burden of illness.

- Health professionals and policy-makers can play important leadership roles in this process at local, national and international levels.

- Answerable objections may be made that this 'integrated' professional regulatory system is elitist and impractical.

- Placing loyalty in action towards the relief of individual patient suffering, rather than achievement of patient 'good', as the primary goal of 'integrated' regulation of medical professionalism is more likely to consistently trigger conscience towards protection of vulnerable patients and to strengthen the general social fabric towards sustainability over millions of years.

Case study: Zeta's story

A teenage girl (Zeta) in an impoverished country went to a New Year's party with a friend. They met a wealthy man who handed them some 'E' and said he could get both girls a job doing exotic dancing in a rich country. Zeta's friend began 'having a wonderful, wild time in her mind', but seemed all right afterwards. She said it was 'like this fantastic journey into the unknown'. So Zeta said, 'All right then, let's have a brew. It was cool. So I went on to "E". The full hap. Started vomiting and apologising to everyone about it. Then I couldn't feel my legs or toes. That was really scary. My friend took me down to the Emergency Department of a private hospital. My new dress was covered in urine and vomit, but they wouldn't see me till they'd checked my insurance status. I told the doctor someone had spiked my drink, 'cause I didn't want the truth written down anywhere, and he said he'd have to report it to the police. The doctor could hardly speak our language. He treated me like a junkie and wanted a bribe before he'd give me any free medicine.'[18] What issues are raised here for an 'integrated' system of medical professional regulation?

Case study: Ben's story

After an arduous process of research and development a new human gene therapy trial is concluded.[19] John, the CEO of the socially conscious corporate manufacturer, seeks 'fast-track' safety, quality, efficacy and cost-effectiveness approval. That process now permits public submissions, one of which states that failure to allow gene therapy may mean the rich can condemn the poor and their children to generations of inequality and hardship.[20] A health minister called Ben decides, in collaboration with his friend John (the CEO), to establish a scheme whereby the new therapy, if approved, will be made available to all citizens below the international benchmark price through a public–private partnership. What issues are raised here for an 'integrated' system of medical professional regulation beyond the age of the market state?

NOTES

Preface

1 Ozdemir, V and Williams-Jones, B (2006) Democracy unleashed – unpacking the Tooth Fairy in drug industry R&D, *Nature Biotechnology* 24(11): 1324–26.

Chapter 1

1 Conference on Security and Cooperation in Europe, *Helsinki Final Act*, 1 August 1975, VII: 'The participating States will respect human rights and fundamental freedoms, including the freedom of thought, conscience, religion or belief, for all without distinction as to race, sex, language or religion. They will promote and encourage the effective exercise of civil, political, economic, social, cultural and other rights and freedoms all of which derive from the inherent dignity of the human person and are essential for his free and full development.'

2 Medical Professionalism Project (2002) Medical professionalism in the new millennium: A physician charter, *Annals of Internal Medicine* 136: 243–48; Freckelton, I (2006) Regulating health practitioner professionalism, in Freckelton, I (ed.), *Regulating Health Practitioners* (Law in Context Series), Sydney: Federation Press, 1–20.

3 Pellegrino, ED and Pellegrino, AA (1988) Humanism and ethics in Roman medicine: Translation and commentary on a text of Scribonius Largus, *Literature and Medicine* 7: 26–31.

4 International Conference on Islamic Medicine, *Declaration of Kuwait*, adopted in 1981 (1401 by the Islamic calendar).

5 Nanji, A (1983) Medical ethics and the Islamic tradition, *Journal of Medicine and Philosophy* 13: 257–62.

6 International Conference on Islamic Medicine, *Declaration of Kuwait*, adopted in 1981 (1401 by the Islamic calendar).

7 Mendelson, D (1998) The medical duty of confidentiality in the Hippocratic tradition and Jewish medical ethics, *Journal of Law and Medicine* 5: 231–38; Rosner, F (1986) *Modern medicine and Jewish ethics*, Ktav Publishing House.

8 Qiu, RZ (1988) Medicine – The art of humaneness: On ethics of traditional Chinese medicine, *Journal of Medicine and Philosophy* 13: 288–94.

9 In a series of cases concerning legislative discrimination against illegitimate children, these courts invoked the *ICCPR* and the *Convention on the Rights of the Child* as aids to constitutional interpretation: 23 June 1993, Tokyo High Court, *Kominshu*, 46, 43; and 5 July 1995, Supreme Court Grand Bench, *Hanrei jiho*, 1540, 3.

10 Grotius, H ([1646] trans FW Kelsey 1995) *De Jure Belli Ac Pacis Libri Tres*, 656 et seq.

11   Carter, KS, Abbott, S and Siebach, JL (1995) Five documents relating to the final illness and death of Ignaz Semmelweis, *Bulletin of the History of Medicine* 69: 255–70.

12   Bell, J (1995) Introduction to the Code of Medical Ethics, in Baker, R (ed.) *The Codification of Medical Morality*, Springer, 65.

13   Osler, W (1991) Aequanimitas, in Reynolds, R and Stone, S (eds) *On doctoring: Stories, poems, essays*, Simon & Schuster, 33–34.

14   Thorwald, J (1961) *The Dismissal: The last days of Ferdinand Sauerbruch, Surgeon*, Thames & Hudson, 43.

15   Women's Cancer Group (1997) Songs of Strength, *Sixteen Women Talk About Cancer*, Macmillan, 55–56.

16   Barr, MD (2001) Medical savings accounts in Singapore: A critical inquiry, *Journal of Health Politics, Health Policy and Law* 26: 709–12.

17   Starfield, B (2005) Insurance and the US health care system, *New England Journal of Medicine (NEJM)* 353: 418–19.

18   Blumenthal, D and Hsiao, W (2005) Privatisation and its discontents: The evolving Chinese health care system, *NEJM* 353(11): 1165–70.

19   Lokuge B, Denniss, R and Faunce, TA (2005) Private health insurance and regional Australia, *Medical Journal of Australia (MJA)* 182(6): 290–93.

20   Sekhon, JS, Reinhardt, UE, Cheng, T, Navarro, V, Tuckson, R, Woolhandler, S, Campbell, T, Himmelstein, DU and Aaron, HJ (2003) Costs of health care administration in the United States and Canada, *NEJM* 349(25): 2461–64. In 1999, health administration costs in the United States were 31 per cent of total expenditure ($1059 per capita), compared with 16.7 per cent ($307 per capita) in Canada. In the United States, the percentage of administrative workers in health care grew from 18.2 per cent in 1969 to 27.3 per cent in 1999; in Canada the number grew from 16.0 per cent in 1971 to 19.1 per cent in 1996: Woolhandler, S, Campbell, T and Himmelstein, DU (2003) Costs of health care administration in the United States and Canada, *NEJM* 349(8): 768–75.

21   Waitzkin, H and Iriart, C (2000) How the United States exports managed care to third world countries, *Monthly Review* 52(1): 1–7.

Chapter 2

1   Pearson, SD, Miller, FG and Emanuel, EJ (2006) Medicare's requirement for research participation as a condition of coverage, *Journal of the American Medical Association (JAMA)* 296 (8): 988–91.

2   *Harper v Baptist Medical Center – Princeton* 341 So 2d 133. See also *Chiasera v Employers Mut. Liability Ins. Co. of Wisconsin* 422 NYS 2d 341, 101 Misc 2d 877 and *Hoesl v US* 451 F Supp 1170, aff 629 F 2d 586 (examinations ordered by insurer and employer respectively).

3   In *Pegram v Herdrich* 530 US 211 (2000), for example, a patient (Cynthia Herdrich) complained of abdominal pain to her physician (Lori Pegram), who was employed under Herdrich's managed care plan with the HMO Carle Clinic Association. Pegram detected signs and symptoms consistent with appendicitis. The HMO, however, had instituted cost-cutting and financial incentive guidelines that encouraged the doctor, instead of ordering an immediate diagnostic ultrasound at a local hospital, to arrange for the

test to be performed eight days later at a more distant health care institution overseen by her employer. In the interim, Herdrich's appendix ruptured, causing peritonitis. The plaintiff sued the HMO for breaching a statutory fiduciary duty, but failed. The HMO's interests immediately rose on the stock exchange.

4   The World Health Organization (WHO), in the Preamble to its Constitution (1946), has termed health 'a state of complete physical, mental and social well being and not merely the absence of disease or infirmity'. This definition has been influential in recent times not only in shifting health policies towards preventive interventions, but also in placing government health responsibilities in a broad social justice context.

5   Ayers, I and Braithwaite, J (1992) *Responsive regulation: Transcending the deregulation debate,* Oxford University Press, 35.

6   Moore, GE ([1903] 1968) *Principia Ethica,* Cambridge University Press, 183–87.

7   Paton, HJ (1948) *The moral law: Kant's groundwork of the metaphysic of morals,* Hutchinson.

8   Probably because this would have offended US policy-makers concerned to preserve national sovereignty in the face of the growing international human rights movement.

9   Rawls, J, Thomson, J, Jarvis, Nozik, R, Dworkin, R, Scanlon, TM and Nagel, T (1997) Assisted suicide: The philosopher's brief, *New York Review of Books* 44(5).

10   Foot, P (1978) *Virtues and vices and other essays in moral philosophy,* Oxford University Press, 2 and 8. See also Pieper, J (1966) *The Four Cardinal Virtues,* University of Notre Dame Press.

11   Kant, I ([trans. Gregor, MJ] 1996) *The Metaphysics of Morals,* Harper & Row, 512.

12   Rawls, J (1976) *A theory of justice,* Harvard University Press, 560; Rawls, J (1980) Kantian constructivism in moral theory, *Journal of Philosophy* 77: 519–26.

13   Pellegrino, ED (1995) Toward a virtue-based normative ethics for the health professions, *Kennedy Institute of Ethics Journal* 5(3): 253–67; Brickhouse, TC and Smith, ND (1997) Socrates and the unity of the virtues, *Journal of Ethics* 1(4): 311–18.

14   Bate, WJ (1977) *Samuel Johnson,* Harcourt Brace Jovanovich, 315.

15   Royce, J (1908) *The Philosophy of Loyalty,* Macmillan, 13–16; Royce, J (1971) The philosophy of loyalty, in Roth, JK (ed.), *The Philosophy of Josiah Royce,* Hackett Publishing Co. Inc., 278.

16   *The World Medical Association: Declaration of Tokyo,* available at http://www.wma.net/e/policy/c18.htm (accessed 14 February 2007).

17   *In the Matter of Karen Quinlan* 70 NJ 10, 355 A. 2d 647 (1976): mandating physician consultation with an 'ethics committee' before deciding to withdraw treatment from a patient in chronic persistent vegetative state.

18   *Canterbury v Spence* 464 F 2d 772 (DC, 1972): developing the legal concept of informed consent.

19   *Roe v Wade* 410 US 113 (1973).

20   Faunce, TA (2005) The UNESCO Bioethics Declaration 'social responsibility' principle and cost-effectiveness price evaluations for essential medicines,

Monash Bioethics Review 24(3): 10–19.

21   Beauchamp, TL (1995) Principlism and its alleged competitors, *Kennedy Institute of Ethics Journal* 5(3): 181–89.

22   The SUPPORT Principal Investigators (1995) A controlled trial to improve care for seriously ill hospitalised patients, *JAMA* 274: 1591–98.

23   Pendleton, D (1983) Doctor–patient communication: A Review, in Pendleton, D and Hasler, J (eds), *Doctor–patient communication*, Academic Press, 5.

24   Meisel, A and Roth, LH (1983) Toward an informed discussion of informed consent: A review and critique of the empirical studies, *Arizona Law Review* 25: 265–346; Katz, J (1977) Informed consent – A fairy tale? Law's vision, *University of Pittsburgh Law Review* 39: 137–45.

25   Faunce, TA (2005) Will international human rights subsume medical ethics? Intersections in the UNESCO Universal Bioethics Declaration, *Journal of Medical Ethics* 31: 173–78.

26   Mertens, T (2003) Nazism, legal positivism and Radbruch's Thesis on statutory injustice, *Law and Critique* 14(3).

27   *Pretty's Case* [2002] 1 FLR 268; *Case of Pretty v UK* (application no. 2346/02).

28   *Judgment No. T-505*, 28 August 1992, Columbian Constitutional Court in (1992) 21 *Revista Mensual Jurisprudencia Doctrina* 1101; *Amparo* action against the Ministry of Health, Supreme Court of Justice, Republic of Venezuela, 9 June 1998.

29   *Minister of Health v Treatment Action Campaign* (2002) Case CCT 8/02.

30   Amnesty International (2004) *Starved of rights: Human rights and the food crisis in the Democratic People's Republic of Korea (North Korea)*, available at: http://web.amnesty.org/library/index/engasa240032004   (accessed 18 February 2007)

31   Farmer, P (2003) *Pathologies of power: Health, human rights and the new war on the poor*, University of California Press; Shaffer, ER and Brenner, JE (2004) International trade agreements: Hazards to health?, *International Journal of Health Services* 34(3): 467–81; Hilary, J (2001) *The wrong model: GATS, trade liberalization and children's right to health*, Save the Children; Angell, M (2005) *The truth about drug companies: How they deceive us and what to do about it*, Random House; Kassirer, JP (2004) *On the take: How medicine's complicity with big business can endanger your health*, Oxford University Press.

32   Drahos, P and Braithwaite, J (2003) *Information feudalism: Who owns the knowledge economy?*, New Press.

33   Article 65(4) allowed developing nations to have a delayed implementation phase, but Article 70(8) allowed patent applications in the interim to be stored in what was termed a 'mailbox'.

34   World Trade Organization (2001) Doha Declaration on the TRIPs Agreement and public health, WT/MIN/(01)/Dec/W/2.

35   Coalition of Service Industries (CSI) (1998) Submission to US Trade Representative (USTR).

36   Pellegrino, ED (1979) Toward a reconstruction of medical morality: The primacy of the act of profession and the fact of illness, *Journal of Medicine and Philosophy* 4(1): 32–41; Pellegrino, ED and Thomasma, DC (1993) *The Virtues in Medical Practice*, Oxford University Press.

37   This is an approach modified from Ayers, I and Braithwaite, J (1992)

Responsive regulation: Transcending the deregulation debate, Oxford University Press.

38   Heisenberg, W ([trans. Pomerans, Arnold J] 1958) *The physicist's conception of nature,* Harcourt, Brace & Co.

Chapter 3

1   Faunce, TA and Gatenby, P (2005) Flexner's ethical oversight reprised? Contemporary medical education and the health impacts of corporate globalization, *Medical Education* 39(10): 1066–74; Faunce, TA (2005) Nurturing personal and professional conscience in an age of corporate globalisation: Bill Viola's 'The Passions', *MJA* 183(11/12): 599–601.

2   Druss, RG (1998) *The magic white coat,* Columbia P&S, 129; Christakis, DA and Feudtner, C (1993) Ethics in a short white coat: The ethical dilemmas that medical students confront, *Academia Medica* 68: 249–56.

3   Students, for example, should bring a high level of critical analysis to any claim that the social responsibility principle in the UNESCO *Universal Declaration on Bioethics and Human Rights* does not actually create a 'principle' that can calibrate legislation or policies produced by the corporate-controlled market state. They should be similarly sceptical of attempts by corporate managers to dimish the importance to medical professionalism of 'soft norms' such as statements in the UNESCO *Universal Declaration on the Human Genome and Human Rights* (1997) that the human genome is the 'heritage of humanity' (Article 1) or that 'the human genome in its natural state shall not give rise to financial gains' (Article 4).

4   Faunce, TA (2003) Normative role for medical humanities, *Lancet* 362: 1859–60.

5   Blythe, R (1981) *The view in winter,* Canterbury Press, 189–90.

6   Stewart, JB (1999) *Blind eye: The terrifying story of a doctor who got away with murder,* Touchstone (Simon & Schuster).

Chapter 4

1   Veatch, RM (1998) Ethical consensus formation in clinical cases, in Have, H and Sass, H (eds) Consensus formation in health care, *Ethics* 17: 24–29.

2   American Medical Association, Code of Medical Ethics E-1.02, available at: http://www.ama-assn.org/apps/pf_new/pf_online?f_n=browse&doc=pol icyfifles/HnE/E-1.02.HTM&&s_t=&st_p=&nth=1&prev_pol=policyfiles/ CEJA-TOC.HTM&nxt_pol=policyfiles/HnE/E-1.001.HTM& (accessed 25 February 2007).

3   British Medical Association, *End of Life Decisions* (1997), available at: http:// web.bma.org.uk (accessed 25 February 2007).

4   Australian Medical Association, Code of Ethics, available at: http://www. ama.com.au/web.nsf/doc/WEEN-6VL8CP (accessed 25 February 2007).

5   Canadian Medical Association, Code of Medical Ethics, available at: http:// www.cma.ca/index.cfm/ci_id/2419/la_id/i.htm (accessed 25 February 2007).

6   Bernstein, H (1978) *No. 46 – Steve Biko,* International Defence and Aid for Southern Africa, 93.

7   Sheldon, T (2003) Drug company employee who queried trial wins appeal, *BMJ* 327: 307.

8   Faunce, T (2004) Developing and teaching the virtue-ethics foundations of health care whistleblowing, *Monash Bioethics Review* 23(4): 41–55.

9   Beecher, HK (1966) Ethics and clinical research, *NEJM* 274(24): 1354–59, reprinted in Kuhse, H and Singer, P (eds) (1999) *Bioethics: An anthology*, Blackwell Publishing Ltd, 421; Annas, GJ and Grodin, MA (eds) (1992) *The Nazi doctors and the Nuremberg Code: Human rights in human experimentation*, Oxford University Press.

10   Weed, DL (1998) Preventing scientific misconduct, *American Journal of Public Health* 88(1): 125–27; Lock, S (1997) Fraud in medical research, *Journal of the Royal College of Physicians of London* 31(1): 90–93; Loff, B and Black, J (2000) The Declaration of Helsinki and research in vulnerable populations, *MJA* 172: 292–96.

11   Wilkinson, M and Moore, A (1997) Inducement in research, *Bioethics* 11(5): 373–76; McNeill, P (1997) Paying people to participate in research: Why not?, *Bioethics* 11(5): 390–94.

12   Shalala, D (2000) Protecting research subjects – what must be done, *NEJM* 343(11): 808–11.

13   Modified from experiences of students at Canberra Clinical School 2002.

14   Kushner, TK and Thomasma, DC (2001) *Ward ethics: Dilemmas for medical students and doctors in training*, Cambridge University Press, 194–95.

Chapter 5

1   Blaylock, D (GAP Communications Director) and Rowley, C (FBI whistleblower) (October 2005) Op-Ed, *New York Times*, available at http://whistleblower.org/content/press_detail.cfm?press_id=322.

2   *Lowns & Anor v Woods & Ors* (1996) *Aust Torts Reports* 81–376, (1995) 36 NSWLR 344, creating a legal obligation on a GP to leave his office and attend a fitting child when summonsed by the child's sister.

3   Amirthalingam, K and Faunce, T (1997) Patching up 'proximity': Problems with the judicial creation of a new medical duty to rescue, *Torts Law Journal* 5: 27–36.

4   Shuman, DW (1993) The duty of the state to rescue the vulnerable in the United States, in Menlowe, MA and McCall Smith, A (eds), *Duty to rescue: Jurisprudence of aid*, Dartmouth Publishing Group, 131; *DeShaney v Winnebago County Department of Social Services* (1982) 489 US 97; Zipursky, B (1990) DeShaney and the jurisprudence of compassion, *New York University Law Review* 65; 1101–29.

5   *Soobramoney v Minister of Health (Kwazulu-Natal)* Constitutional Court of South Africa 27 November 1997, CCT 32/97.

6   *Cattanach v Melchior* (2003) 77 ALJR 1312.

7   *Harriton v Stephens* (2006) 226 ALR 391. The case was heard along with *Waller v James/Waller v Hoolahan* (2006) 226 ALR 457.

8   *Robertson v Nottingham Health Authority* [1997] 8 Med LR 1; *Bull v Devon Area Health Authority* [1993] 4 Med LR 117.

9   Abraham, KS and Weiler, PC (1994) Enterprise, medical liability and the evolution of the American health care system, *Harvard Law Review* 108:

381–98.

10   *Sutcliffe v Jamaica*, HRC comm. 271/1988, UN Doc. A/47/40, annex. IX, SF 246; *Henry and Douglas v Jamaica*, HRC comm. 571/1994, UN Doc. CCPR/C/57/D/571/1994.

11   *Hamel v Malaxos* 25 November 1993, No. 730-32-000370 929 (Québec) (considering provincial human rights legislation).

12   *The Oculist's Case* (1329) LI MS Hale 137(1), fo. 150 (eyre of Nottingham).

13   *Stratton v Swanlond* (Morton's case) YB Hil. 48 Edw. III, fo. 6 pl. 11.

14   *Skyrne v Butolf* (1388) YB Pas 11. Ric II, p. 223, pl. 12; Baker, JH and Milson, SFC (1985) *Sources of English legal history: Private law to 1750*, 362.

15   BGHSt 11 (1958) 111. *Murray v McMurchy* [1949] 2 DLR 442. See also *Hamilton v Birmingham Regional Hospital Board and Keates* [1969] 2 *Br Med J* 456 (sterilisation without consent during caesarean section); *Cull v Royal Surrey County Hospital and Butler* [1932] 2 Br Med J 1195 (patient consented to abortion but hysterectomy performed).

16   *Kerstin v Malmöhus läns Landstingskommun* NJA 1990 442.

17   Katz, J (1984) *The silent world of doctor and patient*, Johns Hopkins University Press, 60–62; Faden, RR and Beauchamp, TL (1986) *A history and theory of informed consent*, Oxford University Press, 145; *Salgo v Leland Stanford jr University Board of Trustees* 317 P 2d 170 (1957).

18   Eser, A (1994) Functions and requirements of informed consent in German law and practice, in Westerhall, L and Phillips, C (eds) *Patient's rights: Informed consent, access and equality*, Nerenius & Santerus, 243.

19   *Walsh v Family Planning Services* [1992] 1 IR 496.

20   *Makino v Red Cross*, Nagoya District Court Judgment, 29 May 1989, *Hanji* 1325, 103, 017; Norio, H (1992) The patient's right to know of a cancer diagnosis: A comparison of Japanese paternalism and American self-determination, *Washburn Law Journal* 31(3): 455–62.

21   *Moore v Regents of the University of California* 793 P. 2d 479, (1990) 271 Cal. Rptr 146.

22   The court in *Truman v Thomas* 27 Cal 3d 285, 611 P 2d 902, (1980) 165 *Cal. Rptr* 308 held that the disclosure duty (that is, risks of no treatment) applied even if the patient refuses the medical procedure and there had been no actual bodily intrusion, thus basing the doctrine on self-determination.

23   *Rogers v Whitaker* (1992) 175 CLR 479 at 490.

24   BGH, 9 December 1958 VI ZR 2033/57 BGHZ 29, 46 (54), cited in Giesen, D (1994) From paternalism to self determination to shared decision making in the field of medical law and ethics, in Westerhall, L and Phillips, C (eds) *Patient's rights: Informed consent, access and equality*, Nerenius & Santerus, 21.

25   A fascinating aspect being that that the initial decision in this tradition of interpretation arose in 1942 while France was occupied by Nazi Germany: Cass req, 28 January 1942 DC 1942.63.

26   In *Rogers v Whitaker* (1992) 175 CLR 479 the Australian High Court stated that the court was the ultimate arbiter of the standard. In *Castell v De Greef* 1994 (4) SA 408 (C) a South African court adopted an informed consent standard very similar to that in *Rogers v Whitaker*. See van Oosten, FFW (1997) Patient rights: A status report on the Republic of South Africa, in Blanpain, B (ed.) *International Encyclopaedia of Laws, World Law Conference:*

Law in motion, Kluwer Law International, 99–109. See the discussion in Giesen, D (1988) *International medical malpractice law: A comparative study of civil liability arising from medical care,* Kluwer Academic, 117–20 and 278–309.

27   *Hollis v Dow Corning Corp & Ors* (1995) 129 DLR (4th) 609 per La Forest J. But see the opposite view, expressed by Sopinka J in the same case, questioning the reliability of the patient's subjective views.

28   Jefford, M, Savulescu, J, Thomson. J et al. (2005) Medical paternalism and expensive unsubsidised drugs, *BMJ* 33: 1075–77.

29   Kennedy, D (1996) *Looking at Shakespeare: A visual history of twentieth century performance,* Cambridge University Press, 171–75, 303 and 304; Kott, J (1966) *Shakespeare our contemporary,* W.W. Norton & Co.

30   Nagel, DC (1988) Human error in aviation operations, in Wiener, EL and Nagel, DC (eds) *Human factors in aviation,* Academic Press; Williamson, AM and Feyer, A (1990) Behavioural epidemiology as a tool for accident research, *Journal of Occupational Accidents* 12: 207–12; Cooper, JB et al. (1978) Preventable anaesthesia mishaps: A study of human factors, *Anaesthesiology* 49: 399–412.

31   *Cannell v Medical and Surgical Clinic* (1974) 315 NE 2d 278 and *McInerney v MacDonald* (1992) 93 DLR (4th) 415 at 424 per La Forest J; *Norberg v Wynrib* (1979) 92 DLR 4th 449; *Emmett v Eastern Dispensary and Casualty Hospital* 396 F 2d 931 (1967).

32   *Breen v Williams* (1996) 186 CLR 71 at 83.

33   Mehlman, MJ (1990) Fiduciary contracting: Limitations on bargaining between patients and health care providers, *University of Pittsburgh Law Review* 51: 365–72.

34   Relman, AS (1980) The new medical-industrial complex, *NEJM* 303: 963–68; Relman, AS (1985) Dealing with conflicts of interest, *NEJM* 313: 749–54; Jenike, MA (1990) Relations between physicians and pharmaceutical companies: Where to draw the line?, *NEJM* 322: 557–63; Chren, MM et al. (1989) Doctors, drug companies and gifts, *JAMA* 262: 3448–52; Daniels, N (1986) Why saying 'no' to patients in the United States is so hard: Cost containment, justice and provider autonomy, *NEJM* 314: 1380–86; Iglehart, JK (1994) The struggle between managed care and fee-for-service practice, *NEJM* 333: 63–68.

35   *Moore v The Regents of the University of California et al.* 793 P 2d 479 (Cal 1990) 482.

36   *Sidaway v Board of Governors of Bethlehem Royal Hospital and Maudsley Hospital* [1985] AC 871904.

37   *Breen v Williams* (1995–96) 186 CLR 71 at 103–05 per Gaudron and McHugh JJ. For a contrary view, see Nourse LJ in *R v Mid Glamorgan Family Health Services; Ex parte Martin* [1995] 1 All ER 356 at 363.

38   *Cour d'Appel de Toulouse* 14 December 1959; *Recueil Dalloz* 1960.1.181; *Revue Trimestrielle de Droit Civil* 1960, 298–99; Giesen, D (1988) *International medical malpractice law: A comparative law study of civil liability arising from medical care,* Kluwer Academic, 12–13.

39   Cross, J (1992) *Shylock: Four hundred years in the life of a legend,* Chatto & Windus.

40   *Moore v Regents of the University of California et al.* 793 P 2d 479 (Cal 1990)

498 per Arabian J.

41   'The human genome in its natural state shall not give rise to financial gains': Article 4 *UDHGHR*.

42   *Tarasoff v Regents of the University of California* 118 Cal. Rptr 129; 529 P2d 553 (1974); 131 Cal. Rptr 14; 551 P2d 334 (1976).

43   *Pate v Threkel* 661 So 2d 278 (Fl 1995).

44   *Safer v Estate of Pack* 677 A 2d 1188 (NJ 1996).

45   *R v Ministry of Defence ex parte Smith* [1996] 1 All ER 257 at 263. Another could be: 'When a fundamental right such as the right to life is engaged, the options open to a reasonable decision-maker are curtailed' (*R v Lord Saville of Newdigate ex parte A* [1999] 4 All ER 860 per Lord Woolf).

46   *Z v Finland* (1997) 25 EHRR 371, (1977) 45 BMLR 107. In *Herczegfalvy v Austria*, however, the European Court of Human Rights adopted a presumption in favour of a psychiatric diagnosis rendering a patient incapable of consenting which contradicts the foundational importance of the ethical principle of patient autonomy: *Herczegfalvy v Austria* A 244 (1992) para 86.

47   *Osman v UK* (1998) 5 BHRC 293; *Palmer v Tees HA* [1999] Lloyd's Rep Med 351, case note by Grubb, A (1999) Med L Rev 331; *Human Rights Act* 1998 (UK).

48   The *Abortion Act* 1967 (UK), for example, has, in section 4, an exception excusing individual medical participation from all but emergency abortions, on grounds of conscientious objection, the burden for proof of which lies on the doctor.

49   Dworkin, R (1993) *Life's dominion: An argument about abortion, euthaniasia, and individual freedom*, Knopf, 11.

50   *Rust v Sullivan* 500 US 173 (1991).

51   *Airedale NHS Trust v Bland* [1993] AC 789, [1993] 2 WLR 316, [1993] 1 All ER 821. *Auckland Area Health Board v AG* [1993] 1 NZLR 235.

52   *Re Quinlan* 70 NJ 10, 355 A 2d 647 (1976); *Superintendent of Belchertown v Saikewicz* 373 Mass 728, 370 NE 2d 417 (1977); *Cruzan v Director, Missouri Dept of Health* 497 US 261 (1990); Gostin, LO (1997) Deciding life and death in the courtroom: From *Quinlan* to *Cruzan, Glucksberg,* and *Vacco* – A brief history and analysis of constitutional protection of the 'right to die', *JAMA* 278(18): 1523–28.

53   *Airedale NHS Trust v Bland* [1993] AC 789, [1993] 2 WLR 316, [1993] 1 All ER 821.

54   *Airedale NHS Trust v Bland* [1993] AC 789 at 864 per Lord Goff of Chieveley.

55   *Case of Pretty v United Kingdom* Application No. 2346/02 para 65.

56   *Mallette v Shulman* (1990) 67 DLR (4th) 321; *Re T (adult: Refusal of Treatment)* [1993] Fam 95; *Airedale NHS Trust v Bland* [1993] AC 789; *Law Hospital NHS Trust v Lord Advocate* 1996 SLT 848.

57   Anonymous (1988) It's over Debbie, *JAMA* 259(2): 272.

58   Gaylin, W, Kass, LR, Pellegrino, ED and Siegler, M (1988) Commentary: 'Doctors must not kill', *JAMA* 259(14): 2139–41.

59   Vaux, KL (1988) Commentary: Debbie's dying: Mercy killing and the good death, *JAMA* 259(14): 2141–42.

60   Proctor, RN (1989) *Racial hygiene: Medicine under the Nazis*, Harvard University Press; Lifton, RJ (1986) *The Nazi doctors: Medical killing and*

the psychology of genocide, Basic Books; Muller-Hill, B (1988) Murderous science, in Annas, GJ and Grodin, MA (eds) (1992) *The Nazi doctors and the Nuremberg Code: Human rights in human experimentation*, Oxford University Press, 17–31.

61   Battin, MP, Rhodes, R and Silvers, A (1999) *Physician assisted suicide: Expanding the debate*, Routledge, 431; Weithman, PJ (1999) Of assisted suicide and the 'philosopher's brief', *Ethics* 109: 548–52.

62   In Australia in 1995 the Northern Territory became the first jurisdiction in the world to decriminalise both physician-assisted suicide and euthanasia, designating both legitimate 'medical treatment': *Rights of the Terminally Ill Act* 1995 (NT). This position was overturned by the *Euthanasia Laws Act* 1997 (Cth), which distinguished euthanasia from withdrawing and withholding treatment, palliative care, the appointment of a health care power of attorney and attempted suicide.

63   Oransky, I (2003) Feeding tube right-to-die case rocks Florida, *Lancet* 362: 1465.

64   *The Limburg Principles on the Implementation of the International Covenant on Economic, Social and Cultural Rights* (1987) UN Doc. E/CN4/1987/17, Principles 26–69.

65   Blendon, RJ, Schoen, C, DesRoches, CM, Osborn, R, Scoles, KL and Zapert, K (2002) Inequities in health care: A five-country survey, *Health Affairs* 21: 182–91; Goldberg, MA and White, J (1995) The relation between universal health insurance and cost control, *NEJM* 332(11): 742–74.

66   Chernichovsky, D (1995) Health system reforms in industrialised democracies: An emerging paradigm, *Milbank Quarterly* 73(3): 339–72.

67   A number of international treaties and declarations have referred to a human right to health or its equivalent, including the *UDHR* (Article 25(1)); the preamble to the influential 1946 *World Health Organisation (WHO) Constitution* adopted by the International Health Conference, New York (19 June–22 July 1946); Article 12(1) *ICESCR;* Article 12 *CEDAW;* Article 24 *CROC;* and Article 5(e)(iv) *Racial Discrimination Convention.* Relevant regional instruments include Article 11 of the *European Social Charter 1961*, Article 16 of the *African Charter on Human and People's Rights 1981* and Article 10 of the *Additional Protocol to the American Convention on Human Rights in the Area of Economic, Social and Cultural Rights 1988*.

68   *Judgment No. T-505*, 28 August 1992, Columbian Constitutional Court in (1992) 21 *Revista Mensual Jurisprudencia Doctrina* 1101.

69   *Soobramoney v Minister of Health* CCT 32/97 27 November 1997, available at http://www.law.wits.ac.za/judgements/soobram.html.

70   *The Limburg Principles on the Implementation of the International Covenant on Economic, Social and Cultural Rights*, UN Doc. E/CN. 4/1987/17, Principle 23.

71   UN Committee on Economic, Social and Cultural Rights, *General Comment No. 14 on the Right to the Highest Attainable Standard of Health in Article 12 ICECSR* e/C.12/2000/4 11/08/2000; Article 12 *ICESCR and* Article 12 *CEDAW;* Eide, A (1987) *UN Sub-Commission for the Prevention of Discrimination and Protection of Minorities, Final Report on the Right to Food,* UN Doc. E/CN 4/Sub. 2 paras 66–69.

72   *Samity v State of West Bengal* (1996) AIR 2426 (Indian Supreme Court),

considering the right to life under Article 21 of the Indian Constitution.

73   *D v UK* European Court of Human Rights, 2 May 1997, 1997-III No. 37; *Sutcliffe v Jamaica* Human Rights Commission, Comm. No. 271/1988 UN Doc. A/47/40.

74   Toebes, B (1999) *The right to health as a human right in international law*, Intersentia, 319–21.

75   *Bill of Rights Act* 1990 (NZ); *Human Rights Act* 2004 (ACT).

Chapter 6

1   *ICCPR Article 7, UDHR Article 5, ECHR Article 3, American Declaration Article XXVI, ACHR Article 5, African Charter Article 5, Torture Convention Article 16, European Convention for the Prevention of Torture and Inhuman or Degrading Treatment or Punishment* signed 26 November 1987 (entry into force 1 February 1989), Doc. No. H (87) 4 1987, ETS 126, repr (1988) 27 *Int'l L Mats* 1152, Article 1.

2   UN High Commissioner for Human Rights (1992) *General Comment 20 on Article 7 ICCPR*, 10/4/1992; Article 53, *Vienna Convention on the Law of Treaties*, adopted 23 May 1969, entry into force 27 January 1980, UN Doc. A/CONF 39/26 repr (1969) 8 *Int'l L Mats* 679; *Barcelona Traction Case* (1970) *ICJ Rep* 2.

3   *The Pinochet Case* [1999] 2 All ER 97, [1999] 2 WLR 827, (1999) 20(1–3) Human Rights LJ 61 at 66 per Lord Browne-Wilkinson, 100 per Lord Millett, 107 per Lord Phillips of Worth Matravers.

4   UN High Commissioner for Human Rights (1992) *General Comment 20 on Article 7 ICCPR*, 10/4/1992.

5   Iacopino, V et al. (1999) *Manual on the effective investigation and documentation of torture and other cruel, inhuman or degrading treatment or punishment (The Istanbul Protocol)*, Physicians for Human Rights, available at http://www.phrusa.org; Moreno, A and Grodin, MA (2000) The not-so-silent marks of torture, *JAMA* 284(5): 538–44; Eisenman, D, Keller, AS and Kim, G (2000) Survivors of torture in a general medical setting, *Western Journal of Medicine* 172: 301.

6   United Nations (1982) *Principles of medical ethics relevant to the role of health personnel, particularly physicians, in the protection of prisoners and detainees against torture and other cruel, inhuman or degrading treatment or punishment*, GA Res. 37/194, 18 December 1982.

7   *Case of D v United Kingdom* European Court of Human Rights, 2 May 1997; Article 3 *ECHR*.

8   Physicians for Human Rights (1994) *Breach of trust: Physician participation in executions in the United States*, Physicians for Human Rights; *Hecker v Chaney* 105 SC 1949 (1985).

9   Amnesty International (1998) *Lethal injection: The medical technology of execution*, Amnesty International, 15.

10   'Sir Richard was also paid a £15,000 fee by the Chemical Manufacturers Association and two other major companies, Dow Chemicals and ICI, for a review that largely cleared vinyl chloride, used in plastics, of any link with cancers apart from liver cancer – a conclusion with which the World Health Organization disagrees. Sir Richard's review was used by the manufacturers'

trade association to defend the chemical for more than a decade': Sarah Boseley (2006) Health Editorial, *The Guardian,* 8 December.

11   United Nations (1999) *Declaration on the rights and responsibilities of individuals, groups and organs of society to promote and protect universally recognized human rights and fundamental freedoms,* GA Res. 53/144, Article 11: 'Everyone who as a result of his or her profession, can affect the human dignity, human rights and fundamental freedoms of others should respect those rights and freedoms.' An example might be doctors becoming involved in the letter-writing campaigns of Amnesty International on behalf of specific unjustly incarcerated individuals.

12   United Nations (1982) *Principles of medical ethics relevant to the role of health personnel, particularly physicians, in the protection of prisoners and detainees against torture and other cruel, inhuman or degrading treatment or punishment,* GA Res. 37/194, 18 December 1982.

13   Geiger, HJ and Cook-Deegan, RM (1993) The role of physicians in conflicts and humanitarian crises: Case studies from the Field Missions of Physicians for Human Rights 1988–1993, *JAMA* 270: 616–25; Gardam, J and Charlesworth, H (2000) Protection of women in armed conflict, *Human Rights Quarterly* 22(1): 148–58; Harvard Study Team (1991) *Report: Health and welfare in Iraq after the Gulf crisis,* Harvard University Press; (1995) *Fourth world conference on women: Action for equality, development, and peace, Beijing Declaration and Platform for Action,* UN GAOR UN Doc. A/Conf. 177/20; Human Rights Watch (1992) *Untold terror: Violence against women in Peru's armed conflict – A report by Americas Watch and Women's Rights Project,* Human Rights Watch; Provost, R (1992) Starvation as a weapon: Legal implications of the United Nations blockade against Iraq and Kuwait, *Columbia Journal of Transnationl Law* 30: 577–83: Committee on the Elimination of Discrimination Against Women ([1990] 1994) *Female circumcision,* General Rec. 14, 9th Sess. 1990, UN Doc. A/45/38/1, *International Human Rights Review* 1: 21–31.

14   Hannibal, K and Lawrence, R (1999) The health professional as human rights promoter: Ten years of Physicians for Human Rights (USA), in Mann, JM, Gruskin, S, Grodin, MA and Annas, GJ (eds) *Health and human rights: A reader,* Routledge, 404; Mann, J (1996) Dignity and health: The UDHR's revolutionary first article, *Health and Human Rights* 3(2): 31; Amnesty International (1996) *Prescription for change: Health professionals and the exposure of human rights violations,* Amnesty International; Adams, V (1998) *Doctors for democracy: Health professionals in the Nepal Revolution,* Cambridge University Press.

15   *Osman v United Kingdom* (ECHR) 87/1997/871/1083, 28 October 1998.

16   Examples relate to *Optional Protocol* to the *ICCPR: International Covenant on Civil and Political Rights* (1966) 999 UNTS 171, entry into force 23 March 1976 (142 ratifications as at 1 January 1999); *Optional Protocol* (1966) 999 UNTS 171, entry into force 23 March 1976 (93 ratifications as at 1 January 1999); the *Declaration Regarding Article 22* of the *Convention against torture and other cruel, inhuman or degrading treatment or punishment* (1984) 1465 UNTS 85, entry into force 26 June 1987 (111 ratifications as at 1 January 1999); and *Declaration regarding Article 22,* entry into force 26 June 1987 (40 declarations as at 1 January 1999). Another may fall under the 1999 *Optional*

Protocol to the Committee overseeing the *Convention on the elimination of all forms of discrimination against women* (1979) 1249 UNTS 13, entry into force 3 September 1981 (163 ratifications as at 1 January 1999), Optional Protocol not yet in force.

17   On 20 June 1859 Henry Dunant, a Swiss businessman, came upon the battlefield of Solferino near the border of his country. Many wounded French and Austro-Hungarian soldiers were dying of neglect. Powerfully motivated by compassion and a sense of injustice, he set aside existing legal principles and political policies and arranged medical assistance for those suffering on either side. Later he argued for an inviolate international convention for impartial protection of wounded in warfare. This became the International Red Cross and the origin of international humanitarian law: McCoubrey, H (1998) *International humanitarian law: Modern developments in the limitation of warfare*, Ashgate Publishing, 16–17.

18   United Nations (1993) *Report of the Secretary-General pursuant to Paragraph 2 of the Security Council Resolution 808*, UN Doc. S/25704 para 35.

19   Sandoz, Y, Swinarski, C and Zimmerman, B (eds) (1987) *International Committee of the Red Cross (ICRC) commentary on the Additional Protocols of 8 June 1977 to the Geneva Conventions of 12 August 1949, ICRC, 147*. These also refer to the World Medical Associations (1962) Rules of medical ethics in time of war and Rules to ensure aid and care for the wounded and sick, particularly in time of armed conflict, ICRC.

20   Hannibal, K (1996) The health professional as human rights promoter: Ten years of Physicians for Human Rights (USA), *Health and Human Rights* 2(1): 111–21 (also in Mann, JM, Gruskin, S, Grodin, MA and Annas, GJ (1999) *Health and human rights: A reader*, Routledge, 404–16).

21   Médecins Sans Frontières developed in 1971 out of dissatisfaction by French physicians with medical relief work in Biafra, when that country was under the influence of the civil war in Nigeria. Médecins du Monde was a 1980s offshoot that occurred as a result of an organisational conflict over chartering a boat to rescue shipwrecked Vietnamese boat people in the South China Sea.

22   Fox, R (1999) Medical humanitarianism and human rights: Reflections on Doctors Without Borders and Doctors of the World, in Mann, JM, Gruskin, S, Grodin, MA and Annas, GJ (eds) *Health and human rights: A reader*, Routledge, 404–16.

Chapter 7

1   Blythe, R (1981) *The view in winter*, Canterbury Press, 136–37, 262.

2   This provided a range of medical services in return for a 50 cents premium per month from lumber mill owners and employees: Mayer, TR and Mayer, GG (1985) HMOs: Origins and development, *NEJM* 312: 590–98.

3   Fox, PD (1996) An overview of managed care, in Kongstvedt, PR *The managed care handbook*, Aspen Publishers Inc., 4–5.

4   Morgenson, G (2006) Fair game: A lump of coal might suffice, *New York Times*, 24 December.

5   Fein, R (1998) The HMO revolution: How it happened and what it means, *Dissent* 45(1): 29–36.

6   Crawshaw, R, Garland, MJ, Hines, B and Lobitz, C (1985) Oregon health decisions: An experiment with informed community consent, *JAMA* 254: 3213–16; Bodenheimer, T (1997) The Oregon Health Plan – Lessons for the nation, *NEJM* 337(9): 651–59.

7   Moynihan, R (2006) Drug giant forks out $65,000 on posh nosh for doctors, *The Australian*, 21 July, available at http://www.theaustralian.news.com.au/story/0,20867,19859691-601,00.html (accessed 22 August 2006).

8   Carreyrou, J (2007) Inside Abbott's tactics to protect AIDS drug: Older pill's price hike helps sales of flagship, *Wall Street Journal*, 3 January, A1.

9   Luce, BR (2005) What will it take to make cost-effectiveness analysis acceptable in the United States?, *Medical Care* 43(7): II 44–48.

10   Faunce, T, Doran, E, Henry, D, Drahos, P, Searles, P, Pekarsky, B and Neville, W (2005) Assessing the impact of the Australia–United States Free Trade Agreement on Australian and global medicines policy, *Globalization and Health* 1: 1–15.

11   Faunce, TA and Buckley, NA (2003) Of consents and CONSORTS: Reporting ethics, law and human rights in RCTs involving monitored overdose of healthy volunteers pre and post the CONSORT guidelines, *Journal of Clinical Toxicology* 41 (2): 93–98.

12   To support life as we know it now, such a new universe would need six conditions of life: 1) a ratio of hydrogen converted to helium in the big bang of 0.007; 2) the electric force divided by the force of gravity at 1036 ; 3) the same relative density of the universe; 4) the same rate of acceleration of the universe; 5) the same amplitude of irregularities in the cosmic microwave bakground radiation; and 6) the same number of spatial dimensions: Rees, M (2000) *Just six numbers: The deep forces that shape the universe*, Basic Books.

13   Midgley, M (2001) Individualism and the concept of Gaia, in Booth, K, Dunne, T and Cox, M (eds) *How might we live? Global ethics in the new century*, Cambridge University Press, 29.

14   Jecker, NS and Jonsen, AR (1995) Health care as a commons, *Cambridge Quarterly of Healthcare Ethics* 4(2): 207; Michels, R (1994) Defining social choices and distributing social resources on the health care commons, *Annals of the New York Academy of Science* 729: 182–89; Buck, S (1998) *The global commons: An introduction*, Island Press; Ostrom, E (1991) *Governing the Commons: The evolution of institutions for collective action (political economy of institutions and decisions)*, Cambridge University Press; Leigh, K (1992) Liability for damage to the global commons, *Australian Year Book of International Law* 14: 129–38; The World Bank (1987) *Financing health services in developing countries: An agenda for reform*, World Bank.

15   *Park v Chessin* (1977) 400 NYS 2d 110, 112.

16   *Smith v Brennano* (1960) 157 A 2d 497 at 503.

17   In the WTO *Canada-Patent Protection of Pharmaceuticals Case*, for instance, the European Community (unsuccessfully) challenged Canadian legislation permitting generic pharmaceutical manufacturers to apply for quality and safety approval before the relevant brand-name patent expires (the 'Bolar exemption'). They were permitted to impugn the legislation as not a 'limited' enough exception to fall within Article 30 of TRIPS, or for being 'discriminatory' as to 'field of technology' under Article 27. A Canadian statute permitting stockpiling of generic drugs in expectation of brand-name patent

expiry, however, was held to be contrary to these TRIPs provisions. That government then risked the threat of trade sanctions if the offending statute was not repealed or amended: *Canada – Patent Protection of Pharmaceutical Products: Complaint by the European Communities* WT/DS114/R (17 March 2000).

18   SCRIP – World Pharmaceutical News, available at http://www.scripnews.com (accessed 14 July 2006).

19   Committee on Economic, Social and Cultural Rights (1995) *Concluding Observations on Philippines,* UN ESCOR, 20 UN Doc. E/C 12/1995/7.

20   Faunce, TA (2006) Towards a treaty on the safety and cost-effectiveness of medicines and medical devices: Protecting an endangered global public good, *Globalisation and Health* 2: 5–18.

21   Kaul, I (2006) Financing global public goods: Challenges, in von Weisacker, EU, Young, OR and Finger, M (eds) *Limits to privatisation: How to avoid too much of a good thing?,* Earthscan, 311.

22   Gilead's effective but also expensive patented medicine for kala-azar, ambisome, was derived from a very toxic drug called amphotericin B, which Gilead scientists inserted into a fat globule, eliminating the toxicity. Professors Shaunak and Brocchini (in partnership with with the Drugs for Neglected Diseases Initiative (DNDi), a not-for-profit organisation linked to Médecins Sans Frontières) now plan to place the drug into sugar-based polymers instead to make it stable in hot climates at 2–3 per cent of the price: Boseley, S (2007) Scientists on a mission to bring cheap drugs to the world's poorest countries, *The Guardian,* 2 January.

Chapter 8

1   Nanotechnology neural implants of a vast range of human knowledge represent possibly the most extreme technology-reductionist way that future leaders of medical professionalism might facilitate this renaissance-type ideal liberal education, with its powerful implications for the training of health professionals and the future of human public health policy development.

2   The resolution arose thanks to persistent and passionate lobbying by Kenya and Brazil, augmented by the input and signatures of 5000 eminent scientists, physicians, policy-makers, Nobel prize winners, members of the European Parliament, and industry representatives.

3   Kelsen, H (1948) Absolutism and relativism in philosophy and politics, *American Political Science Review* 42: 906–12.

4   Locke, J (Laslett, P [ed.] 1967) *Two treatises of government,* Cambridge University Press; Rawls, J (1976) *A theory of justice,* Oxford University Press; Kant, I ([trans. Gregor, MJ] 1999) An answer to the question: What is enlightenment?, in *Practical Philosophy,* Cambridge University Press, 17–18. 'Ideal' does not necessarily mean 'perfect'; an example being the 'ideal' circumstances of moderate scarcity and limited altruism which necessitate the development of principles of justice: Hume, D (1888) *A treatise of human nature,* Hard Press, Bk III, Part II, s.ii, 494–95.

5   Morsink, J (1999) *The Universal Declaration of Human Rights: Origins, drafting, and intent,* University of Pennsylvania Press, 281.

6   Faunce, TA (2004) Developing and teaching the virtue-ethics foundations

of health care whistleblowing, *Monash Bioethics Review* 23(4): 41–55; Faunce, TA (2005) Coherence and health care whistleblowing: A response to Parker, *Monash Bioethics Review* 24(1): 47–49; Palmer, N and Rogers, WA (2005) Whistleblowing in the medical curriculum: A response to Faunce, *Monash Bioethics Review* 24(1): 50–58; Gillett, G (2005) The ethical status of whistleblowers, *Monash Bioethics Review* 24(1): 59–64.

7   Cruess, SR, Johnston, S and Cruess, RL (2002) Professionalism for medicine: Opportunities and obligations, *MJA* 177: 208–10.

8   'The parties' aim in the original position is to establish just and favourable conditions for each to fashion his own unity … given the precedence of right and justice, the indeterminacy of the conception of the good is much less troublesome': Rawls, J (1976) *A theory of justice*, Oxford University Press, 563–64. Norton, D (1973) Rawls' 'Theory of justice': A 'perfectionist' rejoinder, *Ethics* 83: 50–57; Kymlicka, W (1987) Rawls on teleology and deontology, *Philosophy and Public Affairs* 17: 167–76.

9   Dezalay, Y and Garth, B (1996) *Dealing in virtue*, University of Chicago Press; Raz, J (1992) The relevance of coherence, *Boston University Law Review* 72(2): 273–301; Youngs, R (1998) *English, French and German comparative law*, Routledge Cavendish, 40 and 104.

10   'So the portrait of Dr Gachet shows you a face the colour of an overheated brick, burnt by the sun, with red hair and a white cap, against a landscape with a background of blue hills. His clothes are ultramarine, which brings out his face and makes it look pale even though it is brick-coloured. His hands, the hands of an obstetrician, are paler than his face. In front of him on a red garden table are yellow novels and a dark red foxglove flower': *The Letters of Vincent van Gogh* (de Leeuw, R [ed.] 1997), Penguin, 492; Arenberg, K et al. (1990) Van Gogh had Meniere's Disease and not epilepsy, *JAMA* 264: 491–96.

11   Sontag, S (2003) *Regarding the pain of others*, Penguin, 87.

12   de Beauvoir, S (1964) *A very easy death*, Penguin, 51.

13   Cahn, E (1949) *The sense of injustice*, New York University Press; Meron, T (ed.) (1984) *Human rights in international law: Legal and policy issues*, Oxford University Press, vol. 1, 93.

14   Illich, I (1979) *Limits to medicine, medical nemesis: The expropriation of health*, Penguin.

15   Coope, J (1998), *Doctor Chekhov: A study in literature and medicine*, Cross Publishing, 51–53.

16   Bennett, J (1974) The conscience of Huckleberry Finn, *Philosophy* 49: 123–34.

17   Glover, J (1999) *Humanity: A moral history of the twentieth century*, Yale University Press, 150.

18   Donaghy, B (1996) *Anna's story*, Angus & Robertson.

19   Rosenberg, SA (1992) *The transformed cell: Unlocking the mysteries of cancer*, Orion Publishing Co.

20   Watson, J (1999) in panel discussion in Stock, G and Campbell, J (eds) *Engineering the human germline*, Oxford University Press, 73.

FURTHER READING

Angell, M (2005) *The truth about drug companies: How they deceive us and what to do about it*, Toronto: Random House.

Annas, GJ and Grodin, MA (eds) (1992) *The Nazi Doctors and the Nuremberg Code: Human rights in human experimentation*, Oxford: Oxford University Press.

Arendt, H (1973) *The Origins of Totalitarianism*, London: Allen & Unwin.

Bakan, J (2004) *The Corporation: The pathological pursuit of profit and power*, New York: Free Press.

Ball, P (2004) *Critical Mass: How one thing leads to another*, New York: Farrar, Straus and Giroux.

Beauchamp, TL (1995) Principlism and its alleged competitors, *Kennedy Institute of Ethics Journal* 5(3): 181–89.

Beecher, HK (1966) Ethics and clinical research, *New England Journal of Medicine (NEJM)* 274(24): 1354–59.

Blythe, R (1981) *The View in Winter*, Norwich: Canterbury Press.

Booth, K, Dunne, T and Cox, M (2001) *How Might We Live? Global ethics in the new century*, Cambridge: Cambridge University Press.

Cahn, E (1949) *The Sense of Injustice*, New York: New York University Press.

Carruthers, P (2004) *The Nature of the Mind: An introduction*, London: Routledge.

Chalmers, DJ (1996) *The Conscious Mind: In search of a fundamental theory*, Oxford: Oxford University Press.

Chren, MM et al. (1989) Doctors, drug companies and gifts, *JAMA* 262: 3448–52.

Cohen, JC, Illingworth, P and Schuklenk, U (2006) *The Power of Pills: Social, ethical and legal issues in drug development, marketing and pricing*, New York: Pluto Press.

Crawshaw, R, Garland, MJ, Hines, B and Lobitz, C (1985) Oregon health decisions: An experiment with informed community consent, *JAMA* 254: 3213–16.

Daniels, N (1986) Why saying 'no' to patients in the United States is so hard: Cost containment, justice and provider autonomy, *NEJM* 314: 1380–86.

Davies, G (2004) *Economia: New economic systems to empower people and support the living world*, Sydney: ABC Books.

de Beauvoir, S (1964) *A Very Easy Death*, London: Penguin Books.

Drahos, P and Braithwaite, J (2003) *Information Feudalism: Who owns the knowledge economy?*, London: New Press.

Dworkin, R (1993) *Life's Dominion: An argument about abortion, euthanasia, and individual freedom*, New York: Knopf.

Farmer, P (2003) *Pathologies of Power: Health, human rights and the new war on the poor*, Berkeley: University of California Press.

Faunce, TA and Gatenby, P (2005) Flexner's ethical oversight reprised? Contemporary medical education and the health impacts of corporate globalization, *Medical Education* 39(10): 1066–74.

Faunce, TA (2003) Normative role for medical humanities, *Lancet* 362: 1859–60.

—— (2004) Developing and teaching the virtue-ethics foundations of health care whistleblowing, *Monash Bioethics Review* 23(4): 41–55.

—— (2005a) Will international human rights subsume medical ethics? Intersections in the UNESCO Universal Bioethics Declaration, *Journal of Medical Ethics* 31: 173–78.

—— (2005b) Nurturing personal and professional conscience in an age of corporate globalisation: Bill Viola's 'The Passions', *MJA* 183(11/12): 599–601.

Fein, R (1998) The HMO revolution: How it happened and what it means, *Dissent* 45(1): 29–36.

Freckelton, I and Petersen, K (2006) *Disputes and Dilemmas in Health Care*, Sydney: Federation Press.

Glover, J (1999) *Humanity: A moral history of the twentieth century*, New Haven: Yale University Press.

Gostin, LO (2000) *Public Health Law: Power, duty, restraint*, Berkeley: University of California Press.

Heisenberg, W (1958) *The Physicist's Conception of Nature*, London: Hutchinson Scientific and Technical.

Iglehart, JK (1994) The struggle between managed care and fee-for-service practice, *NEJM* 331: 63-68.

Illich, I (1979) *Limits to Medicine, Medical Nemesis: The expropriation of health*, London: Boyars.

Jenike, MA (1990) Relations between physicians and pharmaceutical companies: Where to draw the line?, *NEJM* 322: 557–63.

Kaku, M (2005) *Parallel Worlds: a journey through creation, higher dimensions, and the future of the cosmos*, New York: Doubleday.

Kassirer, JP (2004) *On the Take: How medicine's complicity with big business can endanger your health*, Oxford: Oxford University Press.

Katz, J (1977) Informed consent – A fairy tale? Law's Vision, *University of Pittsburgh Law Review* 39: 137–45.

Kaul, I, Conceicao, P, le Goulven, K and Mendoza, RU (2003) *Providing Global Public Goods: Managing globalisation*, Oxford: Oxford University Press.

Kuhse, H and Singer, P (eds) (1999) *Bioethics: An anthology*, London: Blackwell Publishing Ltd.

Lee K, Buse, K and Fustukian, S (2003) *Health Policy in a Globalising World*, Cambridge: Cambridge University Press.

Linklater, A (1998) *The Transformation of Political Community: Ethical Foundations in the Post-Westphalian Era*, Columbia: University of South Carolina Press.

Mann, JM, Gruskin, S, Grodin, MA and Annas, GJ (eds) (1999) *Health and Human Rights: A reader*, London: Routledge.

Meisel, A and Roth, LH (1983) Toward an informed discussion of informed consent: A review and critique of the empirical studies, *Arizona Law Review* 25: 265–346.

Pellegrino, ED (1995) Toward a virtue-based normative ethics for the health professions, *Kennedy Institute of Ethics Journal* 5(3): 253–67.

Rawls, J, Thomson, J Jarvis, Nozik, R, Dworkin, R, Scanlon TM and Nagel T (1997) Assisted suicide: The philosopher's brief, *New York Review of Books* 44 (5).

Rawls, J (1976) *A Theory of Justice*, Oxford: Oxford University Press.

Relman, AS (1980) The new medical-industrial complex, *NEJM* 303: 963–68.

Relman, AS (1985) Dealing with conflicts of interest, *NEJM* 313: 749–54.

Reynolds, R and Stone, S (eds) (1991) *On Doctoring: Stories, poems, essays*, New York: Simon & Schuster Inc.

Royce, J (1908) *The Philosophy of Loyalty,* Norwood: Norwood Press.

Schachter, O (1983) Human dignity as a normative concept, *American Journal of International Law* 77: 848–53.

Scholte, JA (2000) *Globalization: A critical introduction,* London: Palgrave Macmillan.

Shaffer, ER and Brenner, JE (2004) International trade agreements: Hazards to health?, *International Journal of Health Services* 34(3): 467–81.

Sontag, S (2003) *Regarding the Pain of Others,* London: Penguin Books.

Stewart, JB (1999) *Blind Eye: The Terrifying Story of a Doctor Who Got Away with Murder,* New York: Touchstone (Simon & Schuster).

Stiglitz, J (2006) Scrooge and intellectual property rights, *British Medical Journal* 333: 1279–80.

Stiglitz, J (2006) *Making Globalization Work: The next steps to global justice,* New York: W.W. Norton.

von Weizsacker, EU, Young, OR and Finger, M (2006) *Limits to Privatisation: How to avoid too much of a good thing,* London: Earthscan.

Yunus, M (2005) *Banker to the poor: Micro-lending and the battle against world poverty,* New York: Public Affairs.

INDEX